RECALIBRATING STIGMA

Sociologies of Health and Illness

Edited by
Gareth M. Thomas, Oli Williams,
Tanisha Spratt, and Amy Chandler

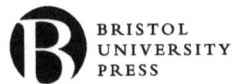

First published in Great Britain in 2025 by

Bristol University Press
University of Bristol
1–9 Old Park Hill
Bristol
BS2 8BB
UK
t: +44 (0)117 374 6645
e: bup-info@bristol.ac.uk

Details of international sales and distribution partners are available at bristoluniversitypress.co.uk

© Gareth M. Thomas, Oli Williams, Tanisha Spratt and Amy Chandler 2025

The digital PDF and ePub versions of this title are available open access and distributed under the terms of the Creative Commons Attribution-NonCommercial-NoDerivatives 4.0 International licence (https://creativecommons.org/licenses/by-nc-nd/4.0/) which permits reproduction and distribution for non-commercial use without further permission provided the original work is attributed.

British Library Cataloguing in Publication Data
A catalogue record for this book is available from the British Library

ISBN 978-1-5292-3582-1 paperback
ISBN 978-1-5292-3584-5 ePub
ISBN 978-1-5292-3583-8 ePdf

The right of Gareth M. Thomas, Oli Williams, Tanisha Spratt, and Amy Chandler to be identified as editors of this work has been asserted by them in accordance with the Copyright, Designs and Patents Act 1988.

All rights reserved: no part of this publication may be reproduced, stored in a retrieval system, or transmitted in any form or by any means, electronic, mechanical, photocopying, recording, or otherwise without the prior permission of Bristol University Press.

Every reasonable effort has been made to obtain permission to reproduce copyrighted material. If, however, anyone knows of an oversight, please contact the publisher.

The statements and opinions contained within this publication are solely those of the editors and contributors and not of the University of Bristol or Bristol University Press. The University of Bristol and Bristol University Press disclaim responsibility for any injury to persons or property resulting from any material published in this publication.

Bristol University Press works to counter discrimination on grounds of gender, race, disability, age and sexuality.

Cover design: SMOJ
Front cover image: UNWANTED

For Lin Codd (Grancha) and
Pauline Thomas (Nan/Grandma Biscuits)

For Roma, Steve, Austin 'Dustbin' West and
his frequently overstimulated mum (OW)

For Betty (TS)

For Robin, and Just Jill (AC)

Contents

Notes on Contributors — vii
Acknowledgements — x

Introduction: Recalibrating Stigma — 1
Gareth M. Thomas, Oli Williams, Tanisha Spratt, and Amy Chandler

1. Stigma, Racism, and Mental Healthcare — 19
   Dharmi Kapadia and Maria Haarmans
2. Stigma and Sexual Arousal: Rethinking HIV-Related Stigma in the Age of PrEP and the Internet — 36
   Jaime García-Iglesias
3. The Contested Nature of Abortion Stigma: From the Individual to the Structural — 52
   Gillian Love
4. Shooting Blanks? Exploring the Assumed Relationship Between Masculinity and Stigma in Male Fertility — 70
   Esmée Hanna, Caroline Law, and Nicky Hudson
5. On the Process of Becoming a Body Fascist: Stigma and Shame in the Moral Economy of Exercise — 87
   Kass Gibson
6. Recalibrating Anti-Stigma: Avoiding Binary Thinking and 'Destigmatisation Drift' in Public Health — 105
   Oli Williams, Amy Chandler, Gareth M. Thomas, and Tanisha Spratt
7. Readdressing Addiction Stigma: Making Space for Being in the World Differently — 123
   Fay Dennis
8. How Stigma Emerges and Mutates: The Case of Long COVID Stigma — 139
   Hannah Farrimond and Mike Michael
9. Notes on a Spoiled Working Identity: Stigma, Illness, and Disability in the Contemporary (Western) Workplace — 156
   Jennifer Remnant

| 10 | Spoiled Identity and the Curated Self: Narrativising Stigma in Parents' Memoirs of Raising Disabled Children
Harriet Cooper | 173 |
| 11 | Studying Up: Understanding Power in Stigmatisation, Discrimination, and Health
Andy Guise, Simone Helleren, and River Újhadbor | 189 |

Recalibrating Stigma: Concluding Thoughts 206
Tanisha Spratt, Amy Chandler, Oli Williams, and Gareth M. Thomas

Index 217

Notes on Contributors

Amy Chandler is Professor of the Sociology of Health and Illness at the University of Edinburgh, UK. She specialises in qualitatively driven studies of mental health, suicide, and self-harm.

Harriet Cooper is Lecturer in Medical Education at Norwich Medical School, UK. She works at the intersection of medical humanities, critical disability studies, and medical sociology, with particular interests in: the figure of the disabled child; auto-ethnography and the uses of lived experience in contemporary culture; shame and stigma; and the material context of knowledge production.

Fay Dennis is Senior Research Fellow in the Department of Sociology at Goldsmiths, University of London, UK. Her research – published in two books and various sociological and drug policy journals – focuses on the socio-material production of illicit and licit drug effects. Fay's current project explores changes and innovations in UK substance use treatment after COVID-19.

Hannah Farrimond is Senior Lecturer in Medical Sociology at the University of Exeter, UK. Her research interests include: stigma theory; pharmaceutical cultures; and the sociology of addiction, in relation to smoking/vaping, alcohol, medications, and psychedelics, among other substances. She published *Doing Ethical Research* with Palgrave in 2012.

Jaime García-Iglesias holds a Chancellor's Fellowship in the Usher Institute at the University of Edinburgh, UK. Jaime has degrees in literature and cultural studies and sociology. His work focuses on the sociology of sexual health as it intersects with technology and sexual and gender minorities.

Kass Gibson is a sociologist and ethnographer based in Newquay, Cornwall, UK. He has an interest in sociologies and histories of sport, physical activity, and health. His research seeks to understand the effects different ways of knowing (past, present, and future) have on how people experience, practice, and understand relationships between being active, their health and wellbeing, and the politics of public health more broadly.

Andy Guise is Senior Lecturer in Social Science and Health at King's College London, UK. His research addresses the health needs and experiences of people who are homeless and using drugs, and the potential for health service and public health responses.

Maria Haarmans is Honorary Research Fellow in Sociology at the University of Manchester, UK, a Trainee Clinical Psychologist at the University of Liverpool, UK, and a member of the ESRC Centre on Dynamics of Ethnicity (CoDE), the UK's largest research centre investigating ethnic inequalities. Her research has focused on gender, psychosis, and ethnic inequalities using methods such as participatory action research.

Esmée Hanna is Reader (Associate Professor) in Health and Wellbeing in Society and a member of the Centre for Reproduction Research at De Montfort University, UK. With a background in sociology, Esmée's research interests are around qualitative psychosocial explorations of gender, health, and the body.

Simone Helleren is Research Associate at King's College London, UK. Simone has worked across the voluntary and statutory sectors with diverse groups focusing on 'involvement and participation' for over 20 years. Her PhD thesis explored engagement with help with young people experiencing homelessness, their support workers, and other significant people in young people's lives.

Nicky Hudson is Professor of Medical Sociology and Director of the Centre for Reproduction Research at De Montfort University, UK. Her research explores experiences of reproductive health and the development and use of a range of reproductive technologies. She has an interest in chronic illness and its management, and especially its intersection with reproductive trajectories.

Dharmi Kapadia is Senior Lecturer in Sociology at the University of Manchester, UK. Her research focuses on stigma, racism, mental health, and older people. She is a longstanding member of the ESRC Centre on Dynamics of Ethnicity (CoDE), the UK's largest research centre investigating ethnic inequalities.

Caroline Law is Senior Research Fellow at the Centre for Reproduction Research, De Montfort University, UK. A sociologist primarily engaged in qualitative research, her research interests centre around reproduction and in/fertility, and particularly their intersections with men and masculinities, families and intimate relationships, reproductive timing, and chronic illness (particularly endometriosis).

Gillian Love is Lecturer in Sociology at the University of Sussex, UK. Her work focuses on the study of reproduction from a feminist and sociological perspective. Her research has focused on a range of reproductive issues including abortion stigma, abortion and class, transgender pregnancy, and parenting during the pandemic.

Mike Michael is a sociologist of science and technology, and Professor of Sociology at the University of Exeter, UK. His research interests include the public understanding of science, everyday life and technoscience, biomedical innovation, and culture. Major publications include *Actor-Network Theory: Trials, Trails and Translations* (Sage, 2017) and *The Research Event: Towards Prospective Methodologies in Sociology* (Routledge, 2021).

Jennifer Remnant is Chancellor's Fellow and THIS Fellow at the Scottish Centre for Employment Research at the University of Strathclyde, UK. Jen's research focuses on the workplace management of long-term ill health and disability.

Tanisha Spratt is Senior Lecturer in Racism and Health at King's College London, UK. Tanisha's research centres on racial inequalities in health outcomes in the UK and the US, and specifically the role of neoliberalism in promoting and sustaining understandings of personal responsibility, deservedness, and grievability with respect to experiences of illness, death, and dying.

Gareth M. Thomas is Reader in the School of Social Sciences at Cardiff University, UK. He is a sociologist with an interest in disability, medicine, health and illness, and reproduction.

River Újhadbor is Research Assistant at King's College London, UK. They are a qualitative health researcher with a background in anthropology, social medicine, and applied theatre. Currently, they are a researcher on the Social Responses to Stigma study, developing a complex systems approach to social exclusion, stigma, and homelessness.

Oli Williams is Lecturer in Co-designing Healthcare Interventions at King's College London, UK. His research focuses on weight-related health, including 'obesity' and eating disorders, stigma, health inequalities, equitable intervention, and participatory research methods.

Acknowledgements

GT

I have benefitted from working with and learning from many colleagues, several of whom have contributed to this book. I am wary of listing them all for fear of forgetting some, though a few deserve a mention. Thanks to Ellie Byrne, Eva Elliott, Janice McLaughlin, Susie Scott, Imogen Tyler, and Elena Vaughan – and the editors and anonymous reviewers at the journals *The Sociological Review*, *Health and Place*, and *People, Place and Policy* – for their respective contributions to my own comprehension of stigma. Imogen: I am so grateful for the invitation to present on the panel 'Rethinking the Sociology of Stigma' at the BSA Annual Conference in 2017, as well as your support of my pursuits since then.

I thank Kayleigh Garthwaite who, in co-organising the workshop 'Stigma, Health and Inequality' with me in 2018, cultivated a space for debating some of the concerns identified within this book. Thanks to Robin Smith for his informative and compelling defence of stigma as an interactional accomplishment. Even where our theoretical commitments might diverge, his insights have been welcome and appreciated. Thanks to my former PhD supervisor and colleague, Joanna Latimer, whose companionship, critical eye, and championing is a gift that I can never properly reciprocate. Given her interest in stigma as a concept, I hope that this collection does her proud.

I thank the Cardiff University School of Social Sciences for providing me with the time and resources to dedicate to this book, as well as running my undergraduate module 'The Sociology of Stigma', which has profoundly shaped my understanding of stigma as a concept over the years. Likewise, I extend my gratitude to the British Academy for awarding me a Mid-Career Fellowship in 2023. Co-writing chapters, and reviewing and editing contributions, for this book were largely undertaken during the fellowship. I am grateful for being afforded the resource to work on my own material, a commodity that I recognise as being so rare and coveted.

Thanks to Amy, Oli, and Tanisha. Writing, reading, and editing can be a solitary affair. Working with them meant that I was collaborating with people who I both respect as scholars and who I consider as friends. I am looking forward to future collaborations with you all!

Thank you to Ellie. Your staunch support of me is always appreciated and never forgotten. I am so fortunate to have you by my side. And thank you to Mabel and Albert, for reminding me of the joy and necessity of a healthy work-life balance. I love you all dearly.

OW

This project has been one of the most fulfilling of my career, and I owe a debt of gratitude to those who made that possible. Gareth, Amy, and Tanisha: I've enjoyed co-editing this book with you so much. It's reminded me how good it can be to work in academia, at a time when I needed reminding. Gareth, I'm so grateful to you for making this happen. I feel very fortunate that when you had this idea you wanted to see it through with me. We're getting dangerously close to being 'old friends' now. I just need to admit to being old enough to have old friends. Amy, after getting so much from your work over the years, it's been great to finally work with you. The conversations we've had while working through ideas for this book, and especially our chapter, have sparked and fuelled so much for me that it won't be long before I'll be trying to convince you to work with me again. So, start preparing your excuses. Tanisha, it's been a lovely way to get to know you. I've got a lot from your insight and energy, so much so that I hope this is the first of many projects we do together. To all the contributors, we took a 'dream team' approach to selecting chapter authors and you haven't disappointed. I've enjoyed and benefitted from working with you all. Thanks for boarding this boat and trusting us with the rudder.

Thanks also to those who have most notably helped me to be in a position to co-edit a book on this topic. I was so fortunate to have been supervised by Ellen Annandale during my PhD. She has always given me so much. John Williams who also supervised my PhD and knew that comparing Nikolas Rose to Philippe Coutinho was what I needed. Those at Loughborough University who changed my life through their teaching and support, principally Alan Bairner, John Evans, Dominic Malcolm, Mike Atkinson, Emma Rich, and Lara Killick. Simone Fullagar, for wanting me in your team and being instrumental in me being awarded the NIHR CLAHRC West Dan Hill Fellowship for Health Equity. Thank you to NIHR CLAHRC West, especially Jenny Donovan, for seeing my potential, and to Dan Hill's family for trusting that my work would honour his memory. Graham Martin for making me his Sandy at SAPPHIRE and supporting me to apply for a THIS Institute Postdoctoral Fellowship. Mary Dixon-Woods for being willing to take a punt on me with that fellowship. Glenn Robert for attempting to wrangle me during my time at King's and helping me end a cycle of precarious employment.

To my given family, Mum, Dad, Ben, Sam, and Joe, and my chosen one, Helen and Austin: this wouldn't have been possible without you. Thanks for supporting and putting up with me.

TS

I am extremely grateful to have benefitted from the wisdom and support of many wonderful colleagues, friends, and family members throughout the time it has taken to edit this book. Firstly, thanks to Gareth, Amy, and Oli for inviting me to co-edit this book while I was still an early career researcher and very much finding my feet. I've learned so much from each of you throughout this whole process, and I'm so grateful for your friendship, guidance, and support. Many thanks to Anne Pollock, Mónica Moreno Figueroa, Hettie Malcomson, Tracey Reynolds, Darin Weinberg, and Laia Bécares for providing the mentorship I needed to dream big and achieve what I would have once thought unachievable. I am grateful to each of you for your encouragement, advice, and support over the years.

Thank you to the Department of Global Health and Social Medicine, King's College London, for affording me the time and resources I needed to complete this book. Thanks also to the Center for Health and Wellbeing, Princeton University, for awarding me a visiting scholarship that allowed me to complete and edit crucial parts of this book. It was truly a privilege to have dedicated writing time to spend on my own research endeavours while I was there, and I am extremely grateful (and lucky!) to have had that opportunity. I began working on this book while I was a lecturer in the School of Humanities and Social Sciences, University of Greenwich, and I am indebted to several colleagues and friends there for their insights and encouragement in its initial stages. Particular thanks to Jessica Simpson, Louise Owusu-Kwarteng, Angus McNelly, Gayle Letherby, and Elena Vacchelli.

Among the many friends who have both supported and inspired me while editing this book, I would like to particularly thank Humaira Chowdhury, Mê-Linh Riemann, Victoria Adams, Ali Meghji, Laura Sochas, Arya Thampuran, and Garima Sahai. You are all incredible scholars and it is such a privilege to both formally and informally learn from you as your careers progress. Thanks to Jihane Boudiaf for all the late night rom-coms, delicious dinners, and hilarious conversations when I've needed them most! You have helped me manage my work-life balance in more ways than you know. Many thanks to my mum and dad for always being ready at the end of the phone to provide a listening ear and sound words of wisdom whenever I start flapping. I love you both very much.

AC

These are brief acknowledgements from me, as I write this from the midst of maternity leave. Thanks principally to my co-editors – Tanisha, Oli, Gareth – it's been a pleasure and a privilege to work with you on this project. I'm especially grateful for the patience and care you've each taken in supporting me to juggle work and family life during the writing and editing of this book!

Further acknowledgements are due to my wonderful colleagues at the Universities of Edinburgh and Lincoln for providing a critical and productive intellectual context in which to do this work – Emily Yue, Alex Oaten, Hazel Marzetti, Ana Jordan, Sarah Huque, Rebecca Helman, and Joe Anderson. Stigma has been an undercurrent in much of the research I've done over the years, and my thinking has grown and evolved over this time thanks to conversations with many people, too numerous to name here. Notable mentions and thanks to: Angus Bancroft, Tineke Broer, Baptiste Brossard, Sarah Cunningham-Burley, Jeni Harden, Ruth Lewis, Tom McGlew (who first started me on my journey into medical sociology), Fiona McQueen, Martyn Pickersgill, Steve Platt, Polly Radcliffe, Zoi Simopoulou, Fiona Stirling, Annie Taylor, and Anne Whittaker.

Final thanks as ever to Jonathan, and our children, for making life outside of work a haven and a joy.

All

This book is the outcome of a joint effort which began in 2021. We were very grateful to receive funding from the Foundation for the Sociology of Health and Illness to organise a two-day workshop ('Recalibrating Stigma') at King's College London, UK, in April 2023. The workshop brought together authors to review, discuss, and refine the brief of the book and content of the chapters. It also included a well-attended seminar with talks from several authors. This was later documented in a co-authored blog in *The Polyphony*. Each of these activities have been joyful and productive, and have fully enriched this collection.

We want to thank each author for their enthusiasm, patience, and engagement throughout the process of producing this book. We appreciated not only their contributions, but their reviews of respective chapters as requested by us. All authors responded thoughtfully and respectfully to this process. We are so pleased with the end result, and we hope that each author is as well. We thank Lee-Ann Ashcroft at Newgen Publishing and the editorial team at Bristol University Press, and in particular Anna Richardson, for their support and patience in seeing this book to completion. Any errors in this book remain our own. Thank you to Joe Williams for bringing the central theme of our book to life in the cover he created for us. Joe co-founded the art collective Act With Love (AWL), who work collaboratively with artists and designers to ensure research can be communicated in accessible and engaging ways in order to help address social justice issues. To see more of this work, visit: www.actwithlove.co.uk. We are also very grateful to The Healthcare Improvement Studies (THIS) Institute for providing funds to pay the open access fee, so that we could ensure that the price of the book was not a barrier to anyone interested in reading it.

Funding

The open access fee for this book was funded by The Healthcare Improvement Studies (THIS) Institute (www.thisinstitute.cam.ac.uk) through a postdoctoral fellowship awarded to Oli Williams (PD-2018-01-001). THIS Institute's mission is to enable better healthcare through better evidence about how to improve.

Introduction: Recalibrating Stigma

Gareth M. Thomas, Oli Williams, Tanisha Spratt, and Amy Chandler

Stigma has long been a central concern for researchers. The concept has travelled across disciplines, accumulating considerable air miles in sociology (and, particularly, in our own specialism of medical sociology/the sociology of health and illness), anthropology, psychology and psychiatry, and public health. As a longstanding theoretical resource, stigma has been a mainstay of research relating to – among other matters – mental health, HIV/AIDS, addiction, obesity, and chronic illness and/or disability. This research tells increasingly familiar tales about the impact of diagnosis and labelling on people's everyday lives and how the stigma of their 'affliction', whatever that might be, negatively affects their wellbeing, interpersonal relationships, and interactions in public spaces. The detrimental impacts of stigma have resulted in professional, private, and public efforts to 'reduce' stigma for certain social groups by, it is claimed, raising awareness and presenting alternative narratives.

Yet, in scholarship on stigma, the term is rarely clearly defined and clarified, and it is often utilised as a vague catch-all term for a range of purported conditions, behaviours, and situations. As the concept is used more and more, it becomes less well-defined and applied. Stigma, Manzo (2004, 413) tells us, is almost never subject to inquiry or overt definition; 'summarising such varied, adaptable, and micro-socially organised behaviour with the "gloss" of stigma fails to capture what actors are actually accomplishing in any context'. It is, for Manzo (2004, 413), one of many 'mundane idealisations' found in the social sciences. A clear example of this is when researchers make assumptions of *what* is stigmatising; for example, it is taken-for-granted that drug use, mental illness, self-harm, 'obesity', HIV/AIDS, and homelessness, as social issues, are held in the unyielding and persistent grip of stigma. Similarly, what stigma *does* is all too often assumed, with researchers commonly failing to explore how and why people's experiences are not uniform.

Stigma, then, is frequently treated as an ever-present feature of an illness or related condition, one which firmly ignites and drives isolation, shame, and exclusion. Smith et al (2022, 891) note how stigma has become a 'catch-all concept for relations between "normal" and "deviant" categories'. It is invoked as an explanation without considering how stigma is produced in actual situations:

> Stigma is treated by social scientists as a thing of the world and, at the same time, a conceptual device for finding order in the world ... It can be found operating as an elevator concept, adding a conceptual lift to mundane observations. Stigma is similarly used as a placeholder concept, marking a conceptual, analytic space without the obligation of filling said space with necessary detail. Stigma is also, we suggest, a bidet concept ... It adds a touch of class, but nobody knows how to use it. (Smith et al, 2022, 891)

This limited precision blunts the analytical potential of stigma as a concept, shrouding more than it informs and, in turn, forcing it to do a lot of heavy lifting (Smith et al, 2022). Stigma is too frequently black-boxed, its inner workings hidden and assumed since it appears to already have a known status which nullifies any challenge to it. This, in turn, dulls a critical analysis of research relating to health, illness, bodies, and medicine. As Prior et al (2003, 219) claimed over twenty years ago: 'Stigma … is creaking under the burden of explaining a series of disparate, complex and unrelated processes to such an extent that the use of the term is in danger of obscuring as much as it enlightens.'

This book, then, seeks to initiate a process of recalibration for the conceptualisation of stigma. It brings together early- and mid-career scholars from the sociology of health and illness who focus on a range of issues commonly associated with stigma, including (but not limited to) mental health, sex, reproduction, 'obesity', eating disorders, self-harm, drug use, COVID-19, chronic illness, and disability. In so doing, the book offers new perspectives to stimulate and intensify conversations around stigma, and to showcase the light that can be shed by studying health and illness sociologically. In a context where the loose use of stigma stifles its explanatory potential, thereby inviting unhelpful and potentially harmful responses or interventions, we argue that recalibrating stigma as a theoretical construct is a worthwhile, and indeed necessary, pursuit.

In this chapter, we outline how sociologists – both within and outside the social study of health and illness – have conceptualised stigma. We begin by returning to Erving Goffman, a sociologist who wrote the classic book *Stigma: Notes on the Management of Spoiled Identity* (Goffman, 1963). Goffman's book is widely regarded as an origin text when it comes to thinking about stigma. He defined stigma as a mark of infamy, disgrace, or reproach which causes shame and embarrassment. However, what is key for Goffman, and is frequently missed when his work is referenced, is how stigma is rooted in interactions and relationships. We argue that this use of Goffman's analysis of stigma – particularly in the sociology of health and illness – often misunderstands, and shows a limited engagement with, his main claims. We agree with Hannem (2022, 51), who suggests that, despite stigma being one of Goffman's most celebrated and well-travelled concepts, it is 'also possibly the most misunderstood and misused in both scholarship and in colloquial discourse'.

In what follows, we turn to recent scholarship on rethinking the sociology of stigma (Scambler, 2018; Tyler, 2020; Tyler and Slater, 2018). This work argues that treatments of stigma in sociology and, particularly, in disciplines such as psychology are dislocated from matters of power, inequality, and structure. Stigma is commonly conceptualised as an individual (behaviour-focused) and apolitical enterprise which cannot be avoided or subverted. Here, we outline the main contentions of such contributions – particularly around the need to recognise and study the political economy of stigma (Tyler, 2020). Moreover, we identify how medical sociology, which is strong on matters of explaining (individual) experiences of health and illness, can be surprisingly weaker on locating these experiences within their wider (structural) contexts.

From here, we outline our priorities for beginning to recalibrate stigma. Drawing upon Hannem (2022, 60), we contend that stigma 'must be understood as operating at both the symbolic (micro) and structural (macro) levels in society'. The book does not provide an overarching definition of stigma for all researchers to work to. The social lives of people do not, and cannot, cleave at neat points; the theoretical devices we use to make sense of people's experiences, equally, must not be rigid and stubborn. Dwelling with the messiness and complexity of people's lives necessitates seeing stigma as a plural, wobbly, contested, and contextual term. It is complexly related to individual and structural factors which are variously entwined, which makes 'simple descriptions, single theories, or straightforward fixes' of stigma ill-advised (Brewis and Wutich, 2019, 19). Recognising this, though, should not give researchers a licence to continue over-using, and avoid defining, stigma. In this book, each chapter – all of which are summarised at the end of this introduction – includes the contributors' explicit attempt to outline their conceptual understanding of stigma and how this relates to their chosen empirical topic. The task of defining stigma, then, is distributed throughout the book.

Erving Goffman on stigma

When reading any social science text on stigma, one is likely to come across a reference to Goffman. Best known for his dramaturgical analysis, Goffman (1963, 1, 5) defined 'the stigmatised' as:

> A blemished person, ritually polluted, to be avoided, especially in public places … While the stranger is present before us, evidence can

arise of [them] possessing an attribute that makes [them] different from others in the category of persons available to [them], and of a less desirable kind – in the extreme, a person who is quite thoroughly bad, or dangerous, or weak. [They are] thus reduced in our minds from a whole and usual person to a tainted, discounted one … [They possess] a stigma, an undesired differentness from what we anticipated.

'The stigmatised' are differentiated from 'the normals' (Goffman, 1963, 5), who do not depart from taken-for-granted expectations of an interactional encounter. However, an important recognition from Goffman is that 'the normal and the stigmatised are not persons, but rather perspectives' (Goffman, 1963, 138). Stigma is not a *trait* which belongs to a person or group. Rather, stigma is accomplished within interactions. This is why, for Goffman, face-to-face interaction is the prime scene of analysis – and stigma occurs when normative expectations which steady and sustain the interaction order are breached. For Goffman (1963, 32), anticipating this means people internalise judgements relating to 'the standards against which they fall short'. People are, therefore, self-conscious and calculated in their interactions; they are always 'on' (Goffman, 1963, 26).

Goffman claims that this interactional dance is shaped by whether a person's attributes are public knowledge ('discredited') or concealable ('discreditable'). A discreditable status, for Goffman (1963, 42), invites serious interactional management; a person must consider whether 'to display or not to display, to tell or not to tell, to lie or not to lie, and in each case, to whom, how, when and where'. Goffman (1963, 19) also suggests that people, whether their status is discredited or discreditable, might find 'sympathetic others' who 'adopt [their] standpoint in the world' and 'share with [them] the feeling that [they are] human and "essentially" normal'. This can be both persons who share the same status ('the own') or someone who may not share the same status, but accepts them ('the wise'). Both groups, Goffman (1963, 30) says, can feel a 'courtesy stigma', in which people are stigmatised by association (for example, a family member or partner). Regardless of the form that stigma takes, Goffman (1963, 146) says that his arguments can apply across multiple people and groups: '[S]tigmatized persons have enough of their situations in life in common to warrant classifying all these persons together for purposes of analysis'.

Beyond Goffman?

Despite being influential and extremely well-cited, Goffman's work on stigma has been subject to critical scrutiny (Kusow, 2004). For example, within disability studies, while some scholars positively reflect on Goffman's analysis (Brune and Garland-Thomson, 2014; Love, 2021; Healey and Titchkosky, 2022), others are vocally critical of his approach (Fine and Asch, 1988; Gleeson, 1999; Grinker, 2020). This critique includes perceptions of Goffman's: detached and othering tone; disregard of the historical and political origins of stigma; assumption of disability *as* deviance; dismissal of what is meant by 'norms'; lack of theorising around agency, resistance, and power; focus on 'management', leaving an unjust world intact, and; dislocation of stigma from broader social contexts.

Such charges are reflected in more recent sociological scholarship (Tyler, 2020) and in the social study of health and illness. For example, Scambler (2004, 2018) critically reflects on his own earlier use of stigma (Scambler and Hopkins, 1986) as giving epistemic authority to the biomedical perspective, aligning with a deficit/impairment-focused understanding of disability, and assuming a passive tone associated with victimhood. He suggests moving beyond individualistic, Goffman-inspired conceptions of stigma and, instead, analysing structures of power and the possibility of resistance to stigma. Likewise, Charmaz (2020, 22) reassesses Goffman's concept of stigma and suggests placing stigmatising experiences relating to illness and disability 'in larger structural perspectives, policies, and practices dominated by neoliberalism'. Farrugia (2009, 1012) also claims that, while Goffman's conceptualisation is still the main theoretical foundation for studies of stigma in medical sociology, this scholarship rarely considers the origins of negative stereotypes, frequently positions the stigmatised as powerless victims, and fails to consider 'structural power relationships'. Similarly, while using Goffman's work in his research on weight stigma and masculine identities, Monaghan (2017, 2022) claims any analysis of stigma must move beyond Goffman by examining macro-social relations as well as neoliberal ideology and scapegoating.

Reinterpreting Goffman

While there is validity to all these critiques, it has not been sufficiently acknowledged that scholars within and outside of medical sociology are often guilty of misinterpreting and misrepresenting Goffman's position. Scambler (2004, 29) himself reflects on this, claiming that the sociology of chronic illness and disability often references Goffman's work in a 'ritualistic' rather than 'sustained' manner. There is an insufficient attempt to refine and revise Goffman's assertions. Instead, the tendency is to *cite-and-write*. Goffman's work is cited because it is *the* text to cite, but his conceptualisation of stigma is subsequently engaged with in only a cursory manner.

Many scholars have interpreted Goffman's treatment of stigma 'more concretely', that is, as 'objectively present and more or less visible' (Charmaz, 2020, 22). Stigma, in turn, is presented as an accessory attached to identities and/or attributes. However, Goffman (1963) wrote that stigma is based in interaction. Related to an argument that we made earlier in the chapter, researchers often incorrectly treat stigma as an '*a priori* category, based on taken-for-granted assumptions about what attributes are devalued' (Hannem, 2022, 52). Such an understanding suggests a misconception of Goffman's work. It is assumed that Goffman proposes a permanence to stigma which creates an unbridgeable division between 'the stigmatised' and 'the normals'. Yet, Goffman was clear that these are not *persons*, but *perspectives*; they are normative ideals 'against which almost everyone falls short at some stage in [their] life' (Goffman, 1963, 128). Goffman's point is we can all momentarily experience stigma, we all have something that discredits us, and we all engage in stigma management at some point in our lives – though this will be a more permanent task for some than it is for others: 'Stigma involves not so much a set of concrete individuals who can be separated in two piles, the stigmatized and the normal … [It is] a pervasive two-role social process in which every individual participates in both roles' (Goffman, 1963, 137–8).

A further criticism of Goffman is that he too readily discards power and structure. Tyler (2020) charges his analysis with being too conformist and conservative, as maintaining the (inequitable) status quo, and as solidifying the position of those subject to stigma (see also Link and Phelan, 2014). However, for Müller (2020), Goffman appreciated people's place in the social structure, and how the contingencies people encounter in interactions must be understood in relation to 'the history, the political development, and the current policies of the [stigmatised] group' (Goffman, 1963, 138). It was, Müller argues, simply not his main interest. Goffman was aware of the structural antecedents of stigma, but his analysis of them was absent due to his focus being on the minutiae of everyday life and individuals' anticipation of stigma and presentation of self. Strong (1983, 352) also notes how Goffman recognised the capacity for individuals to pursue their own interests, purposes, and identities. Similarly, Goffman does touch on power in other contributions, such as *Asylums* (Goffman, 1961). While he may rarely use the term *power* in that book, he describes how institutions strip people of individual identity markers and cause them to suffer a 'personal defacement' (Goffman, 1961, 18). He reminds us that the self 'is not a property of the person to whom it is attributed, but dwells rather in the pattern of social control that is exerted in connection with the person by [them] and those around [them]' (Goffman, 1961, 168).

These arguments are presented not to doggedly defend Goffman or to discount the (several legitimate) critiques of his scholarship. Rather, they highlight the folly in critiquing Goffman for misunderstandings or misapplications of his work and to ensure that this does not lead to the baby being thrown out with the bathwater. There is value in recognising stigma as a 'phenomenon of interaction order' (Smith et al, 2022, 890) and incorporating this *within* – rather than discarding it for – analyses focused on power and structure. Nonetheless, in recent years, the emphasis in sociology on stigma has been the 'macro' (rather than 'micro') properties of stigma. This considerable shift in focus is summarised in the next section.

Stigma power

There has been a resurgence of sociological work on stigma in recent years (Parker and Aggleton, 2007; Scambler, 2009, 2018; Tyler, 2020; Tyler and Slater, 2018). In two well-cited accounts, Link and Phelan (2001, 2014) argue for a post-individualist analysis of stigma. They consider how stigma relates to exploitation, control, and exclusion, and how it is exercised through (visible/invisible) cultural distinctions of value and worth. For Link and Phelan, stigma only occurs when labelling, stereotype, and separation join in ways that create negative material consequences:

> Stigmatisation is entirely contingent on access to social, economic, and political power that allows the identification of differentness, the construction of stereotypes, the separation of labelled persons into distinct categories, and the full execution of disapproval, rejection, exclusion, and discrimination ... We apply the term stigma when elements of labelling, stereotyping, separation, status loss, and discrimination co-occur in a power situation that allows the components of stigma to unfold. (Link and Phelan, 2001, 367)

Tyler's (2020) recent work on the machinery of stigma similarly makes a point of taking power seriously. A critic of Goffman's early formulation of stigma, Tyler (2020, 7) also charges the social sciences more broadly with neglecting stigma as a vehicle of power and violence, and how it is 'propagated as a governmental technology of division and dehumanisation'. Tyler critiques passive psychological scholarship on, for instance, self-stigma and the internal emotional and cognitive processes of affected individuals. For Tyler (2020, 8), therefore, emphasising structural arrangements over individual behaviour means researchers can go beyond 'individualistic, ahistorical, and politically anaesthetised conceptualisations' of stigma. This locates stigma, instead, in a political register, that is, as embedded in capitalist relations and a form of violence that causes social and political injuries. This comprehension of stigma also involves attending to how stigma emerges *from above* (including in political rhetoric and media and policy discourse) and along classed, racialised, nationalist, and gendered lines. Stigma machines, Tyler says, move and morph depending on the systems they are designed in, and the desires of those who design them. Stigma, then, is orchestrated to enable, reproduce, and normalise inequalities.

Scholarship on rethinking the sociology of stigma is still growing at the time of writing, though some researchers in the social study of health and illness have picked up on similar imperatives (Scambler, 2018; Monaghan, 2022). For example, Metzl and Hansen (2014, 127) identify how public health, social science, and critical race studies scholars have started to 'locate stigma not just in the attitudes of individual persons, but in the actions of institutions, markets, and health care delivery systems'. In their analysis of stigma and global health, Brewis and Wutich (2019) identify how stigma is an effective political tool for oppressing certain populations and reinforcing the status quo in ways that make resistance difficult. In her research on mental illness, Kapadia (2023) argues that stigma operates against a backdrop of structural and institutional racism in ways that shape access to treatment.

Recent attempts to revisit and reconceptualise stigma have clearly been valuable and well-received in various quarters, including in some of our own scholarship (Williams and Annandale, 2019, 2020; Chandler, 2020; Thomas, 2021; Dolezal and Spratt, 2023) and, as will become clear, in this book. However, at the same time, we must avoid an unnecessary binary. A recent dominance of structural analyses of stigma can be seen to relegate and diminish the centrality of the interaction order. There is no need for scholars to erect strict battlelines between *individual* (/interactionist) or *structural* approaches to the study of stigma. There is a need for both; neither focus should overshadow the other. What is important is recognising that if either is detached from the other, this produces only a partial analysis of stigma.

Recalibrating stigma: 'micro' and 'macro'

Debates on stigma are often polarised by an emphasis on 'structural' or 'interactionist' approaches. *But can we do both?* The risk in devoting oneself to either approach in isolation is that conversations are siloed; debates become insular without recognising the potential value of cross-pollination. This is not to denounce purists. A monogamous commitment to the principles of a theoretical field (for example, interactionism) can be apposite and understandable, depending on the empirical topic. Yet, it can also limit our outlook and blunt the analytic potential of a concept like stigma, and the impact an analysis of stigma might otherwise have. There is a need to move away from singular, blinkered explanations that emphasise micro *or* macro approaches as *the* way to conceptualise stigma.

This book sets out from the position that analyses of how stigma plays out in people's everyday lives (that is, seeing stigma as embedded in the interaction order) are enhanced by a critical engagement with notions of power, history, inequality, and structure. This is where popular attempts to revitalise a sociology of stigma (Link and Phelan, 2014; Scambler, 2018; Tyler, 2020) are helpful. As Pescosolido (2015) says, an interactionist (micro) conceptualisation of stigma – focused on people's everyday experiences – is apt, but this should be complemented by other theoretical and empirical contributions. According to Hansen et al (2014, 77), this means appending a more 'macro' dimension to a comprehension of stigma by 'linking local, interpersonal strategies for managing identities and social value to larger institutional processes of the State, the exercise of power, class relations, and cultural and ideological impositions of meaning and value'. Doing this allows for a more dynamic analysis engaging both structure and experience – where experience informs a structural analysis, and vice versa (McLaughlin, 2017). But *how* might this be done? Hannem's (2012, 2022) arguments are valuable in this respect. Hannem (2022, 60) suggests merging a micro (Goffman-inspired) insight with a historical (Foucault-inspired) approach to highlight the relationship between power, knowledge, and stigma:

> Stigma must be understood as operating at both the symbolic (micro) and structural (macro) levels in society. The macro functions of structural stigma serve as a form of legitimation for the control of populations that have been deemed undesirable or as a threat to the dominant group and its norms. Symbolic and structural stigma exist as a feedback loop in neoliberal society in which symbolic devaluation and discredit of stigmatised categories legitimises increasingly intrusive forms of surveillance, intervention, and control on its members – who are most often marginal.

This approach is consistent with Tyler's (2020) recent work on the machinery of stigma as a strategy of government and control. However, this framing is, for Hannem (2022), a useful extension, rather than a dismissal, of an interactionist conceptualisation of stigma. It means we can situate everyday interactions and experiences of stigma in the structural contexts that mould them. Only focusing on the micro risks ignoring the structures of power and knowledge that shape interactions, and only focusing on the macro risks ignoring the lived experiences of marginalised people and failing to fully recognise the effects of stigma. Marrying both these perspectives is crucial to confront popular trends in stigma studies that presume the existence of stigmatised categories (thus putting the theoretical cart before the horse) and disregard how society brands and excludes people in ways which are inseparable from cultures and histories of violence, trauma, and marginalisation. This also means considering how stigmatising processes, which must not be seen as universal and inevitable, play out for different people in different ways in different social situations. We can consider, for example, practices of intra- and inter-stigma *within* groups of persons where stigma is thrusted onto *Others*, that is, where people slaughter Others to avoid their own social death (Thomas, 2016).

Researchers should both clarify what they mean by stigma and recognise that its interpretation and effects are not universal. Too often, stigma is treated as an adhesive device unanimously attached to entire categories of people, intimating a form of passivity whereby labels are determinative and inflexible. Stigma and power are seen to be of inverse proportions, so stigma victimises those identified (including, on occasion, by sociologists themselves) as powerless (Manzo, 2004; Müller, 2020). The notion that people passively accept a stigmatised status and adapt to this may not represent people's experiences (Millen and Walker, 2001).

There must be a recognition, in turn, of how people might subvert and rework stigma. When researchers have examined this, they regularly do so through a lens of management and coping strategies, such as attempts to 'pass' (Goffman, 1963) by concealing (stigmatising) information from other people. Resistance to stigma is analysed at an individual level; a single person labours to maintain their identity in the face of negative stereotypes (Hannem, 2012). A structural appreciation of stigma is helpful here for chipping away at the foundations of people's unfair and problematic assumptions. Taking fat activism as an example, Monaghan (2017) claims that thinking of resistance in a structural way addresses the ineffectiveness of identity politics which, while vital for elevating lived experiences and rethinking cultural representations, only goes so far. For instance, efforts to redefine fatness as 'acceptable or a badge of pride, rather than a mark of disgrace', are welcome, but may not be 'socially transformative and liberating for most people medically labelled overweight or obese' (Monaghan, 2017, 193).

However, others suggest that any robust appreciation of stigma resistance must also be attentive to more mundane practices of resistance in everyday life – while simultaneously being alive to how a person's agency to resist stigma can be bounded and located in contexts of material and structural constraint (Sebrechts, 2023; Thomas, 2024). Put simply, the 'same' stigmatising status can have different impacts owing to people's differing socioeconomic and sociocultural circumstances. This is how stigma can further marginalise certain groups and exacerbate inequalities. It is much easier for someone to *shake it off* if, in other aspects of their life, their value is assumed and/or they have the comforts afforded by affluence. However, stigma can be compounding if a person has other features in their life that leaves them vulnerable to marginalisation and compromises their capacity to resist stigma. Whatever form that an analysis of stigma resistance takes, it should foreground 'the individual and collective voices of those who are usually silenced' (Hannem, 2012, 26).

Book structure

This book has eleven chapters covering a diverse range of issues. In Chapter 1, 'Stigma, racism, and mental healthcare', Dharmi Kapadia and Maria Haarmans consider the relationship between mental illness stigma and institutional racism. They contemplate how mental illness narratives about racially marginalised groups have surfaced and endured in ways that continue to shape mental healthcare pathways. Drawing on interviews with racially marginalised people with severe mental illness, Kapadia and Haarmans attend to two intertwined systems of power: racism and stigma. They recognise how some people lament their mistreatment within mental health services, yet they were unable to tease out whether this is based on the grounds of race, their mental illness, or both. Other participants recognised how their treatment was informed by racist assumptions and stereotypes communicated by healthcare providers. Kapadia and Haarmans argue for recalibrating the popular comprehension of mental illness stigma to challenge conventional understandings, in which disadvantage is racialised.

In Chapter 2, 'Stigma and sexual arousal', Jaime García-Iglesias explores the experiences of 'bugchasers' – a heterogenous group of gay men who eroticise HIV – and suggests that they offer an inroad for examining how HIV-related stigma is navigated. Deviating from scholarship which frames stigma exclusively as a blockage to HIV treatment and prevention, García-Iglesias explores how, while stigma is felt by many bugchasing men, they also recognise the pleasures, arousals, and desires associated with HIV. Theorising the meaning of stigma for these men, García-Iglesias problematises orthodoxy around HIV-stigma by arguing that the eroticising of HIV and its prevention are not mutually exclusive. Moreover, the resignifying of HIV as stigmatising *and* arousing is shaped using pre-exposure prophylaxis (PrEP) and the internet. To fully understand stigma, García-Iglesias says, we must understand the transformative role that both technologies have had in HIV and sexuality more broadly, and the role of arousal and pleasure in people's experiences and perceptions of HIV.

In Chapter 3, 'The contested nature of abortion stigma', Gillian Love maps recent conceptual developments with respect to how abortion is stigmatised. Love critiques psychological and quantitative framings of stigma as a static attribute possessed by, or imposed on, women choosing to abort a pregnancy. Attending to stigma as power, Love proposes four interrelated approaches – discursive, intersectional, biopolitical, and embodied – for understanding abortion stigma. While examining the discursive character of abortion reveals its unstable and contested nature, an intersectional understanding places it within contexts of marginalisation through the axes of gender, race, class, and disability. Moreover, a biopolitical analysis involves considering the nation-building and nationalist imaginaries of abortion, while the embodied character of abortion demonstrates the interconnection of political discourse with fleshy bodies.

In Chapter 4, 'Shooting blanks?', Esmée Hanna, Caroline Law, and Nicky Hudson provide an overview of the literature on male in/fertility. They start by addressing the assumption that men who are infertile feel, and must navigate, stigma on account of associations between (hegemonic) masculine norms and being both virile and fertile. In this comprehensive summary, Hanna and colleagues show how research on male infertility fails to engage with stigma in a meaningful way. Stigma is, simply, assumed. Hanna and colleagues go on to recognise the cultivation of 'new' masculinities that are presumed to result in less stigma for men. Conversely, they suggest that research, including their own, indicates that men conforming to 'new' masculinities continue to reference the shame and stigma of infertility. As such, Hanna and colleagues call for more substantive and theoretically informed empirical work on men's experiences of infertility – with stigma being one possible theoretical resource to do this.

Kass Gibson, in Chapter 5, 'On the process of becoming a body fascist', examines the role of exercise and physical activity in shaping our understandings of morality and how, specifically, imperatives to *move more* reinforce stigma as an embodied process. Drawing on Norbert Elias' figurational sociology, Gibson frames stigma as a process whereby experiences of power inferiority are interpreted as individual inferiority. He argues that stigma is an inherent aspect of contemporary exercise practices. Two emotional responses – embarrassment and shame – are connected to stigma via what he calls the moral economy of exercise (with exercise being a rather recent invention) and the concept of 'body fascism' (how bodies are viewed as objects with the role of maximising productivity and minimising disease risk through being fit). Gibson claims that this analysis helps us to understand how being *physically fit* has become conflated with being *morally fit*.

In Chapter 6, 'Recalibrating anti-stigma', we – Oli Williams, Amy Chandler, Gareth Thomas, and Tanisha Spratt – argue that recalibrating stigma should involve recalibrating *anti*-stigma. By revisiting the ethics of stigma in public health, we illustrate how the moral certainty evident in the pro-/anti-stigma lobbies obstructs an acknowledgement and understanding of the complexity, inconsistency, and diversity of stigma and its effects. Using the example of anti-stigma efforts in the field of mental health, we propose a novel concept – 'destigmatisation drift' – to explain how approaches to anti-stigma can weaken efforts to address social drivers of suffering, illness, and stigma. We continue our exploration of the tensions in anti-stigma theory and practice through the examples of 'obesity', anorexia, and self-harm. Each case captures how complicated the moral and practical considerations of addressing stigma are, and why an oversimplistic pro-/anti-stigma framing is an inadequate route to understanding or addressing these issues.

Fay Dennis, in Chapter 7, 'Readdressing addiction stigma', tells the stories of people using drugs. Drawing on Goffmanian and Deleuzo-Guattarian insights, her research prompts a recalibration of stigma to ponder how people who use drugs are 'blocked' in their ability to 'be in the world'. Stigma is conceived of by Dennis as relational; people are constrained by their association with addiction and drug use in ways that prevent them from living full lives. Dennis distinguishes this argument from anti-stigma work which attempts to disentangle stigma from addiction and, even, uses the (pathological) narrative of addiction to destigmatise people who use drugs. In shifting the problem of drugs from the drug or person using them to the environment in which they operate, Dennis reconfigures drug use or addiction, instead, as ways of people being in the world differently. This more hopeful narrative seeks to open up possibilities for people who use drugs to be accepted and to inhabit identities more easily alongside 'drug user' or 'addict'.

Chapter 8, 'How stigma emerges and mutates', by Hannah Farrimond and Mike Michael, traces the empirical complexities of long COVID stigma. Drawing on Farrimond's theory of 'stigma mutation', Farrimond and Michael conceptualise how stigma emerges and changes over time (or mutates) in three ways: 1) 'lineage' (how stigma becomes connected to other stigmas and histories of stigma); 2) 'variation' (how stigma changes emerge in relation to differing environments and cultures); and 3) 'strength' (how stigma intensifies or weakens over time). The authors extend this definition by recognising how these dimensions are intertwined in both predictable (or what they call 'territorialised') and unpredictable (or what they call 'de-territorialised') ways. Their analysis suggests a picture of stigma as a shifting array of interrelations. This conceptualisation is attuned to the possibility that stigma might alter in complex, and not always predictable, ways in the future.

Jennifer Remnant's contribution in Chapter 9, 'Notes on a spoiled working identity', discusses the experiences of disabled workers and workers with long-term health conditions or symptoms (such as chronic pain, leakiness, and fatigue). Remnant suggests that these 'unruly bodies' require management – such as concealment or disclosure – in the workplace, with varying effects. Claims of ill-health and disability, Remnant says, risk being dismissed as disingenuous or indicative of poor work performance. Informed by this knowledge, stigma informs workers' relationships (at work) and negotiations of legitimacy, deservingness, and performance. The bodies of ill and disabled workers, Remnant suggests, challenge the social organisation of workplaces that are built on unobtainable ideals exaggerated under neoliberal rule and associated competition and managerialism.

In Chapter 10, 'Spoiled identity and the curated self', Harriet Cooper examines memoir culture and how parents of disabled children articulate narratives that are designed to dismantle notions of loss, misfortune, and stigma. Cooper says that memoirs, together with reinforcing dominant deficit-focused disability scripts, can hinder the emergence of a more transformative and macrosocial conceptualisation of stigma. In her analysis, Cooper assumes a materialist concept of stigma, recognising how stigma arises in a network of unequal class and power relations. Using this definition, along with the scholarship of Puar (2017) and Berlant (2008), Cooper argues that the conventions of life-writing promote overly individualist conceptualisations of stigma, where disability – in this case – is framed as something to navigate and overcome. Simply telling stories cannot, Cooper says, connect with wider political goals. The chapter concludes with Cooper encouraging researchers working on stigma to consider and spell out the political economy of cultural production.

Andy Guise, Simone Helleren, and River Újhadbor begin Chapter 11, 'Studying up', with a nod towards recent scholarship that urges researchers to study the institutional actors playing key roles in manufacturing and maintaining stigma. Treating stigma as a process defined by power and inequality, rather than a fixed property of an individual or group, Guise, Helleren, and Újhadbor offer an account of how researchers working on the social study of health and illness might 'study up' on stigma. They outline three essential ingredients for this: 1) 'power' (there is a need to identify what power is and how it plays out for people); 2) 'positionality' (there is a need to know how researchers who are studying up shape and limit what can be studied); and 3) 'practice' (there is a need to figure out what methods can be used to study power). They summarise three case studies to exemplify these imperatives: transmedicine and 'evidence-based' care; place-based stigma and urban regeneration; and leprosy workers and the power of claims to stigma. They conclude with reflections on what studying up on stigma can productively bring to health and illness research.

Finally, we conclude the book with a short chapter that attempts to tease out how and why recalibrating stigma is so vital, and the various issues that need to be considered within any future sociological research on the interplay of health, illness, and stigma.

Conclusion

This introduction has provided an account of how stigma has been theorised within the social sciences, and why it is now necessary to recalibrate stigma. The plurality of perspectives in this book makes it clear that there is not one way to define and analyse stigma. The book points to the many ways that it can be defined and analysed, though this chapter suggests marrying 'micro' and 'macro' understandings of stigma is a productive way forward. Our intention, instead, is to emphasise the value and obligation of clarifying concepts (stigma, in this case) and what we mean by them in the research we do. Our hope is that this collection rescues what is submerged in current treatments of stigma in the social study of health and illness (and beyond). We expect the audience for this book to be researchers in the social sciences along with health and social care practitioners, policy makers, and other stakeholders.

All chapters end with several bullet-point recommendations (under the heading '*Could things be different?*') to show how understanding and approaching stigma differently could improve research, policy, practice, and people's everyday lives. This is because we hope this collection can offer practitioners, activists, and other interested readers new ideas and directions to inform how they understand and address stigma. Whoever chooses to pick up this book, we want them to see it as an energising and provocative resource for thinking through, and applying, new conceptualisations of stigma. We would also like it to be seen as a book that shows how sociological analyses of stigma can contribute to positive change in society.

References

Berlant, L. (2008) *The Female Complaint: The Unfinished Business of Sentimentality in American Culture*, Durham, NC: Duke University Press.

Brewis, A. and Wutich, A. (2019) *Lazy, Crazy, and Disgusting: Stigma and the Undoing of Global Health*, Baltimore: Johns Hopkins University Press.

Brune, J. and Garland-Thomson, R. (2014) 'Forum introduction: Reflections on the fiftieth anniversary of Erving Goffman's *Stigma*', *Disability Studies Quarterly*, 34(1).

Chandler, A. (2020) 'Shame as affective injustice: Qualitative, sociological explorations of self-harm, suicide and socioeconomic inequalities', in M.E. Button and I. Marsh (eds), *Suicide and Social Justice: New Perspectives on the Politics of Suicide and Suicide Prevention*, London: Routledge, pp 32–49.

Charmaz, K. (2020) 'Experiencing stigma and exclusion: The influence of neoliberal perspectives, practices, and policies on living with chronic illness and disability', *Symbolic Interaction*, 43(1): 21–45.

Dolezal, L. and Spratt, T. (2023) 'Fat shaming under neoliberalism and COVID-19: Examining the UK's Tackling Obesity campaign', *Sociology of Health and Illness*, 45(1): 3–18.

Farrugia, D. (2009) 'Exploring stigma: Medical knowledge and the stigmatisation of parents of children diagnosed with autism spectrum disorder', *Sociology of Health and Illness*, 31(7): 1011–27.

Fine, M. and Asch, A. (1988) 'Disability beyond stigma: Social interaction, discrimination, and activism', *Journal of Social Issues*, 44(1): 3–21.

Gleeson, B. (1999) *Geographies of Disability*, London: Routledge.

Goffman, E. (1961). *Asylums: Essays on the Social Situations of Mental Patients*, New York: Vintage Books.

Goffman, E. (1963) *Stigma: Notes on the Management of Spoiled Identity*, New York: Penguin.

Grinker, R.R. (2020) 'Autism, 'stigma', disability: A shifting historical terrain', *Current Anthropology*, 61(S21): 55–67.

Hannem, S. (2012) 'Theorizing stigma and the politics of resistance: Symbolic and structural stigma in everyday life', in S. Hannem and S. Bruckert (eds), *Stigma Revisited: Implications of the Mark*, Ottawa: University of Ottawa Press, pp 10–28.

Hannem, S. (2022) 'Stigma', in M.H. Jacobsen and G. Smith (eds), *The Routledge International Handbook of Goffman Studies*, London: Routledge, pp 51–62.

Hansen, H., Bourgois, P. and Drucker, E. (2014) 'Pathologizing poverty: New forms of diagnosis, disability, and structural stigma under welfare reform', *Social Science and Medicine*, 103: 76–83.

Healey, D. and Titchkosky, T. (2022) 'A primal scene: disability in everyday life', in M.H. Jacobsen and G. Smith (eds), *The Routledge International Handbook of Goffman Studies*, London: Routledge, pp 242–52.

Kapadia, D. (2023) 'Stigma, mental illness and ethnicity: Time to centre racism and structural stigma', *Sociology of Health and Illness*, 45(4): 855–71.

Kusow, A.M. (2004) 'Contesting stigma: On Goffman's assumptions of normative order', *Symbolic Interaction*, 27(2): 179–97.

Link, B.G. and Phelan, J.C. (2001) 'Conceptualizing stigma', *Annual Review of Sociology*, 27(1): 363–85.

Link, B.G. and Phelan, J.C. (2014) 'Stigma power', *Social Science and Medicine*, 103: 24–32.

Love, H. (2021) *Underdogs: Social Deviance and Queer Theory*, Chicago: University of Chicago Press.

Manzo, J.F. (2004) 'On the sociology and social organization of stigma: Some ethnomethodological insights', *Human Studies*, 27(4): 401–16.

McLaughlin, J. (2017) 'The medical reshaping of disabled bodies as a response to stigma and a route to normality', *Medical Humanities*, 43(4): 244–50.

Metzl, J.M. and Hansen, H. (2014) 'Structural competency: Theorizing a new medical engagement with stigma and inequality', *Social Science and Medicine*, 103: 126–33.

Millen, N. and Walker, C. (2001) 'Overcoming the stigma of chronic illness: Strategies for normalisation of a "spoiled identity"', *Health Sociology Review*, 10(2): 89–97.

Monaghan, L.F. (2017) 'Re-framing weight-related stigma: From spoiled identity to macro-social structures', *Social Theory and Health*, 15: 182–205.

Monaghan, L.F. (2022) 'Goffman and medical sociology', in M.H. Jacobsen and G. Smith (eds), *The Routledge International Handbook of Goffman Studies*, London: Routledge, pp 171–83.

Müller, T. (2020) 'Stigma, the moral career of a concept: Some notes on emotions, agency, Teflon stigma, and marginalizing stigma', *Symbolic Interaction*, 43(1): 3–20.

Parker, R. and Aggleton, P. (2007) 'HIV-and AIDS-related stigma and discrimination: A conceptual framework and implications for action', in R. Parker and P. Aggleton (eds), *Culture, Society and Sexuality: A Reader*, London: Routledge, pp 459–74.

Pescosolido, B.A. (2015) 'Erving Goffman: The moral career of stigma and mental illness', in F. Collyer (ed), *The Palgrave Handbook of Social Theory in Health, Illness and Medicine*, London: Palgrave Macmillan, pp 273–86.

Prior, L., Wood, F., Lewis, G. and Pill, R. (2003) 'Stigma revisited, disclosure of emotional problems in primary care consultations in Wales', *Social Science and Medicine*, 56(10): 2191–200.

Puar, J. (2017) *The Right to Maim: Debility, Capacity, Disability*, Durham, NC: Duke University Press.

Scambler, G. (2004) 'Re-framing stigma: Felt and enacted stigma and challenges to the sociology of chronic and disabling conditions', *Social Theory and Health*, 2(1): 29–46.

Scambler, G. (2009) 'Health-related stigma', *Sociology of Health and Illness*, 31(3): 441–55.

Scambler, G. (2018) 'Heaping blame on shame: "Weaponising stigma" for neoliberal times', *The Sociological Review*, 66(4): 766–82.

Scambler, G, and Hopkins, A. (1986) 'Being epileptic: Coming to terms with stigma', *Sociology of Health and Illness*, 8(1): 26–43.

Sebrechts, M. (2023) 'Towards an empirically robust theory of stigma resistance in the "new" sociology of stigma: Everyday resistance in sheltered workshops', *The Sociological Review*, 72(5): 1117–35.

Strong, P.M. (1983) 'Review essay – the importance of being Erving: Erving Goffman, 1922–1982', *Sociology of Health and Illness*, 5(3): 345–55.

Smith, R.J., Atkinson, P. and Evans, R. (2022) 'Situating stigma: Accounting for deviancy, difference and categorial relations', *Journal of Evaluation in Clinical Practice*, 28(5): 890–6.

Thomas, G.M. (2016) '"It's not that bad": Stigma, health, and place in a post-industrial community', *Health and Place*, 38: 1–7.

Thomas, G.M. (2021) 'Dis-mantling stigma: Parenting disabled children in an age of "neoliberal-ableism"', *The Sociological Review*, 69(2): 451–67.

Thomas, G.M. (2024) '"We wouldn't change him for the world, but we'd change the world for him": Parents, disability, and the cultivation of a positive imaginary', *Current Anthropology*, 65(S26): S32–54.

Tyler, I. (2020) *Stigma: The Machinery of Inequality*, London: Zed Books.

Tyler, I. and Slater, T. (eds) (2018) *The Sociological Review Monographs: The Sociology of Stigma*. London: Sage.

Williams, O. and Annandale, E. (2019) 'Weight bias internalization as an embodied process: Understanding how obesity stigma gets under the skin', *Frontiers in Psychology*, 10: 953.

Williams, O. and Annandale, E. (2020) 'Obesity, stigma and reflexive embodiment: Feeling the "weight" of expectation', *Health*, 24(4): 421–41.

1

Stigma, Racism, and Mental Healthcare

Dharmi Kapadia and Maria Haarmans

Introduction

Ethnic inequalities in mental healthcare are a longstanding major problem in the UK, with little improvement in the mental healthcare experiences of ethnic minority people in the past five decades (Keating, 2002; Kapadia et al, 2022). Compared to white people, Black people are four times as likely to be compulsorily detained in a psychiatric unit (Halvorsrud et al, 2018). Further, people from Black, South Asian, and Chinese backgrounds are less likely to be offered talking therapies, and more likely to be subjected to intrusive treatments such as injectable anti-psychotic medication (Das-Munshi et al, 2018). Mental illness stigma has been theorised as a driving factor in these inequalities, with suggestions that stigma inhibits help-seeking, which results in ethnic minority people using mental healthcare when they are in crisis, leading to negative trajectories of treatment (Memon et al, 2016). The UK Department of Health and Social Care (2021, 90) have stated there is a lack of engagement with services by ethnic minority people due to 'perceptions held within their communities for example around recognising mental health problems early, on levels of associated stigma, as well as a distrust of services'. Institutional racism (Macpherson, 1999) has also been shown to be a fundamental driver of ethnic inequalities in mental healthcare (Fernando, 2017).

However, the ways in which mental illness stigma and institutional racism are interconnected has not been considered. Specifically, an examination of how narratives about mental illness stigma in ethnic minority groups may themselves have been shaped by institutional racism is absent from the field. The poor mental health of many ethnic minority people and their subsequent inadequate, and often harmful, mental healthcare (Nazroo et al, 2020) drives the necessity to critically evaluate the way in which mental illness stigma narratives about ethnic minority populations have surfaced, developed, and endured, and how they shape mental healthcare pathways (Kapadia, 2023).

In this chapter, we call for a recalibration of how mental illness stigma is understood in relation to ethnic minority people and their mental healthcare, pushing beyond stereotypical, racialised notions of mental illness stigma that have come to prevail in the field. We use in-depth interview data from a research project with ethnic minority people with severe mental illness to interrogate how mental illness stigma and institutional racism operate in mental healthcare.

Background

Mental illness stigma, according to the World Psychiatric Association (2019), is the 'single most important barrier to quality of life of mental health consumers and family members'. The damaging nature of stigma was further consolidated in the Lancet Commission on Ending Stigma and Discrimination in Mental Health (Thornicroft et al, 2022, 1438), which stated that mental illness stigma 'contravene[s] basic human rights and [has] severe, toxic effects on people with mental health conditions that exacerbate marginalisation and social exclusion'. However, the workings of mental illness stigma are not well understood in relation to ethnic minority people and their mental healthcare.

In the UK, there seems to be widespread support (in academic literature, mental health practice, and policy) for the notion that there is greater mental illness stigma in ethnic minority groups (referring largely to Black African, Black Caribbean, Pakistani, Indian, Bangladeshi, and Chinese people) than the White British population. The thesis tends to be that, *culturally*, there is more stigma in these groups due to certain religious, spiritual, or traditional beliefs about mental illness and the stigma that seeking help for these problems engenders (Shefer et al, 2013). This supposed greater level of mental illness stigma in ethnic minority populations is said to deter help-seeking, and ultimately lead to more severe mental illness and poorer mental health outcomes (Campbell and Mowbray, 2016).

These explanations are prevalent among healthcare professionals, charities, and advocacy groups working with ethnic minority groups, as well as people who are suffering, or who have suffered, with mental illness and their family members. The UK Department of Health and Social Care (2021) White Paper, *Reforming the Mental Health Act*, placed stigma in ethnic minority groups as one of the reasons for ethnic inequalities in mental healthcare pathways. This is one example of how debates in this area have placed mental illness stigma at the forefront of explanations for the deep ethnic inequalities we see in access to, and experiences of, mental health services. Furthermore, these explanations label ethnic minority people not only as *the stigmatised* but also as *the stigmatisers*. This is in line with how all people with mental illness are labelled: both as the victims of stigma and situated as part of the general public that hold stigmatising attitudes (Pescosolido and Martin, 2015). This ignores how social structures produce and strengthen stigmatising attitudes and the ways those in powerful social roles (such as mental healthcare professionals) can stigmatise others to a greater extent than those with less power (Link and Phelan, 2014).

The evidence behind this focus on stigma in ethnic minority groups is limited. Two systematic reviews (Eylem et al, 2020; Misra et al, 2021) show there is some evidence that mental illness stigma is greater in ethnic minority groups compared to white majority groups, although the difference (statistical effect size) is small. Further, almost all qualitative studies in the field (for a review, see Kapadia, 2023) sample *only* ethnic minority participants (with no white comparison sample). As such, claims about mental illness stigma being particularly problematic for ethnic minority groups, and as something that is more instrumental in mental healthcare pathways for these groups, is largely unsubstantiated. These studies have compounded the racialisation that ethnic minority people are already subjected to by implying that a person's ethnic minority status and their *culture* are the reasons for mental illness stigma (Kapadia and Bradby, 2021). This is similar to the racialisation processes that are seen in explanations for mental illness in ethnic minority groups; erroneous arguments are made that heavily imply that there is something innate within ethnic minority groups that causes mental illness – namely, that simply belonging to a certain ethnic group can explain illness (Kapadia and Bradby, 2021). In terms of mental illness stigma, ethnic minority people are blamed for their poor mental health. The implication is that stigma has impeded their help-seeking, meaning that they have not received appropriate mental health treatment at the right time which has, in turn, worsened their mental health. Importantly, stigma is not argued to operate in the same way for people from White backgrounds. Indeed, their ethnic background is not proposed to be the reason for stigma in these groups.

Stigma definitions in previous studies vary greatly, although conceptualisations tend to fall into four key categories, drawing on the work of Goffman (1963), Corrigan et al (2014) and Pescosolido and Martin (2015): 1) public stigma (stereotypes, prejudice, and discrimination enacted by the general public); 2) self-stigma (internalised acceptance of stereotypes and prejudice); 3) courtesy stigma, also known as affiliative stigma or stigma by association (stereotypes, prejudice, and discrimination experienced by people associated with a person who has mental illness); and 4) structural stigma (stereotypes, prejudice, and discrimination embedded into laws, policies, and practices, and enacted predominantly by public institutions).

Tyler and Slater (2018, 732) have argued for a more sophisticated analysis of power in stigma, and its impact on reproducing inequalities, through focusing on 'stigma as a political apparatus' as well as the role of social structures (such as institutions and the State) in the construction of hegemonic discourses. This coalesces with calls in the field to move away from using public, self-, and courtesy stigma as primary explanations for inequalities in mental health, and to focus more on structural stigma (Hatzenbuehler, 2016). Structural stigma is often not measured in quantitative surveys, nor has it been considered in many qualitative studies. Consequently, there has been little consideration of how stigma embedded in laws, policies, and organisations impacts on ethnic minority people's mental healthcare pathways. This underlines the limitations of empirically studying the effects of structural stigma without a methodological approach that centralises the role of institutions.

Further, the relationship between structural stigma and institutional racism in the psychiatric and psychological professions has not been sufficiently examined. Institutional racism is defined here as discriminatory policies and norms embedded in large institutions (such as the National Health Service [NHS]) and captures a broad range of practices that perpetuate differential access to services and opportunities within institutions. This is distinguished from structural racism, which refers to broader processes embedded in the make-up of societies and governments that lead to disadvantage for ethnic minority people in accessing economic, physical, and social resources. Both types of racism are different from interpersonal racism, which is defined as discriminatory treatment during personal interactions, such as verbal or physical abuse, but also refers to acts of ignoring or avoiding people due to their ethnic background. Previous attempts to theorise the 'double stigma' (Gary, 2005) – also referred to as intersectional stigma (Turan et al, 2019) – of mental illness and racism have not attempted to explain and understand what it means to be marginalised within these two systems, or how multiple aspects of a person's social identity (for example, ethnic background, gender, sexuality, disability status, poverty status) can compound and worsen inequalities (Taylor and Richards, 2019; Turan et al, 2019). Specifically, there has been no consideration of how institutional racism shapes both the experiences of mental illness stigma and the narratives about the effects of mental illness stigma on mental healthcare pathways in ethnic minority groups.

A thorough investigation of the similarities between the two systems of power (stigma and racism), how they relate to each other, and how both negatively impact on ethnic minority people is required to understand ethnic inequalities in mental healthcare. An explanation that connects structural stigma and institutional racism is vital considering the racism that ethnic minority people face seeking help for mental illness and in their subsequent mental health treatment (Kapadia et al, 2022).

In the remainder of this chapter, we demonstrate the complexities of how mental illness stigma is experienced by ethnic minority people with severe mental illness, particularly focusing on the stigma enacted by health and social care staff working in institutions, and how experiences of being stigmatised are difficult to separate from experiences of racism and racialisation.

Data and methods

We use data from the Synergi Collaborative Centre Participatory Action Research project. Synergi was a five-year research programme to rethink and transform understandings of ethnic inequalities in severe mental illness and mental healthcare. We undertook in-depth qualitative interviews guided by participatory research action methodology (Haarmans et al, 2022), to understand the life-course experiences of ethnic minority people with severe mental illness (defined here as any form of psychotic disorder).

To be eligible, participants had to be aged 18 years or over and identify as being from an ethnic minority background and as having a severe mental illness. Participants were recruited purposively via contact with a range of voluntary, community, and social enterprise organisations in the Greater Manchester (UK) area. The final sample size was 22 participants. We interviewed 12 women, nine men, and one person identifying as non-binary; participants' ages ranged from 22 to 63 years. Participants came from a range of Black (N=10: Black British, Black Caribbean, Black African), South Asian (N=7: South Asian, Pakistani, Indian, Kashmiri, Punjabi) and Mixed (N= 5: Mixed White and Black, Mixed White and Asian) ethnic backgrounds. The descriptors used for ethnic background are those that were stated by participants; they were only changed for participants where it was deemed that participants' stated ethnic backgrounds, along with the data presented in this chapter, may put them at risk of identity disclosure. More than three quarters of the sample were born in the UK (N=17, 77 per cent) and those who had migrated to the UK from other countries (N=5, 23 per cent) had done so as young children or teenagers.

The biographical narrative interpretive method (Wengraf, 2001) was chosen to conduct individual interviews with participants, to elicit life stories, particularly focusing on participants' experiences of racism in mental health services. The interview consisted of three 'sub-sessions', which were used to interview participants over the course of one or two interviews. In sub-session one, interviewers asked one question (a single question inducing narrative [Wengraf, 2001]) and gave participants an hour to give their life stories. Interviewers asked follow-up questions (sub-session two), based on the narrative in sub-session one, phrasing the questions using the participant's own words. In sub-session three, interviewers asked any remaining questions that were relevant for answering the research questions that had not been covered in sub-sessions one or two.

The project adopted a participatory research action framework (Gaventa and Cornwall, 2008), which aims to involve people that are affected by the research problem under investigation (racism in mental health services) in all stages of the research. The research team consisted of four academic researchers and five co-researchers; the latter identified as being from an ethnic minority background and as having lived experience of severe mental illness and were recruited as researchers to the project based on these criteria (for more detail on our experience of working within a participatory action research framework, see Haarmans et al, 2022). The team conducted interviews between October 2019 and October 2020. All names used in this chapter are pseudonyms. Ethical approval for the study was granted by the University Research Ethics Committee at the University of Manchester.

Joint analysis sessions were held with the aim of foregrounding the co-researchers' insights considering their subjectivity and lived experiences of mental illness and of the mental health system. We coded the data using reflexive thematic analysis (Braun and Clarke, 2021), particularly focusing on experiences of stigma and racism, in the context of seeking, and receiving, services to help with mental health problems. The results are organised into three themes: 1) myth-busting stigma narratives; 2) stigma experienced at the hands of statutory institutions; and 3) disentangling stigma and racism.

Results

Myth-busting narratives of mental illness stigma

Within participants' narratives, we found some reference to stigmatising views held about mental illness within their communities. In several cases, this was not linked to, or used as an explanation for, either a worsening of mental illness or as a major factor in not seeking help for a mental health problem. Rather, participants gave examples of how mental illness was viewed negatively within communities that they felt a part of, and how this had sometimes meant that they were treated without sufficient understanding by their families or people in their social network due to their mental illness. Sunita talked about the secrecy surrounding mental illness in her family, referring both to her own mental illness and that of her family members:

> I think being Asian and … being Muslim as well having these ideas of it being to do with the devil or, I don't know, fear. There's a lot of secrecy around it, it was always very hush-hush, you didn't tell people that this was going on, there was no support from the partners of the ones who had it. So, for example, my Mum, she didn't really get any support from the rest of the family, and it was always just this thing

that was kept on the quiet ... I suppose they didn't want people to be embarrassed, they didn't want people to think there's a crazy person in the family, sort of thing. (Sunita, 42 years old, female, Indian)

Where stigma was used as an explanation for why help had not been sought from mental health services, reasons given by participants sometimes mimicked dominant narratives that were prevalent about stigma in ethnic minority groups (Kapadia, 2023). However, on a deeper analysis of these narratives, we found that reasons for a lack of help-seeking were more complicated. Marcia talked about her mother not seeking help on her behalf when she was self-harming at a very young age, and attributes this to the shame that would ensue from 'the community' and the church. However, later in her interview, Marcia explained that her mother was complicit in the physical and sexual abuse that she was subjected to, which is likely an equally strong, if not stronger, factor in her mother's decision not to get help for Marcia's problems:

That's where I started my first psychiatric input at [very young age] because I was cutting and the school intervened. I think if school hadn't, my Mum wouldn't have because back then, it was never, it was more taboo to have mental health issues, it was even more taboo to not be right in the head. So, to have a psychiatrist come in and see your child, and if that got out into the community, 'will that get out into the church?' Oh god, no. You go to extraordinary lengths to prevent that from happening [because] it brought such a shame on the family, on the community and on the church ... I've been told by multiple therapists over the years ... because of the beating I suffered in childhood and, as a result of things like having my bones broken so early and so consistently, I developed a tolerance for pain. So, the thing with my mother is she's that sadistic that if she was beating you, she wouldn't stop unless she either saw blood or she heard a bone break. (Marcia, 47 years old, female, Black Caribbean)

For some participants, the stigma they experienced from friends, family, and members of their wider communities was not viewed as related to their ethnic background, or the ethnic background of friends and family. Instead, participants explained that the stigma experienced due to their mental illness was symptomatic of overarching discourses of mental illness and derogatory views held by the public, often in relation to particular diagnoses. Further, it was evident from participant narratives that they themselves often did not hold stigmatising views about mental illness. Charlie talked about being misunderstood and shunned due to their mental illness, and how they experienced stigma from others as uncaring and unsympathetic:

I feel that people don't take you seriously like, you know, when I took all those pills, I felt that people just thought I was silly and impulsive, you know, like a silly little girl taking all these pills. There was no, 'why did you do this?' There was no caring response. It was just a bit crap, and I really struggle when people are shouting [at] me. I just cower and cry and can't handle it … All I needed really was a hug, to be honest, and again it just makes me feel like people don't know me. They don't know how to treat me and, again, that misunderstood feeling. (Charlie, 26 years old, non-binary, Black British)

Stigma experienced at the hands of statutory institutions

Many participants recounted their experiences of being stigmatised by psychiatrists, mental health nurses, psychologists, and social workers (all people working in statutory institutions) during assessment and treatment for mental illness. These stigmatising experiences in hospitals, therapy rooms, and their own homes permeated the narratives of our participants, and affected their mental health and the quality of care that they received. Importantly, experiences of stigma from healthcare professionals were evident in more than half of the participants' accounts, suggesting this was not a rare occurrence, but rather something that was commonplace in encounters with health and social care services.

Participants talked about being stigmatised by psychiatrists and social workers based on their diagnosis of personality disorder (Trevillion et al, 2022), with presumptions made about prognosis in terms of ability to work, recover, and have meaningful relationships (Bonnington and Rose, 2014; Sheehan et al, 2016). This was evident in the interview with Sohal, who talked about the dehumanising treatment and the overriding message that he would not recover from his mental illness:

My early days of mental health services was very poor. They ran like institutions. You weren't seen as a human being or a young person. It was almost like you were seen as someone who had mental health issues and just seen as a diagnosis in that view and the rest did not matter. So, in the early days, it was very institutionalised, very regimented, very kind of, 'you're not well and you're never going to be well'. (Sohal, 43 years old, male, Pakistani)

The power of institutions to reproduce hegemonic discourses that lead to discriminatory practices is further evident in Kamran's narrative. He described how it was not only white mental health staff, but also staff from racialised backgrounds, who internalised dominant biogenetic discourses regarding psychosis that led to non-collaborative approaches to care, particularly the administration of psychotropic medication:

> Their attitude generally around speaking to me, around giving medication, they would speak very little. And these were people from, who could speak my language, people from BME [Black and minority ethnic] communities ... They had very stigmatising and very outdated attitudes, and there was a lot of stigma and discrimination around your mental health. (Kamran, 30 years old, male, South Asian)

Previous research has demonstrated how anti-stigma campaigns promoting biogenetic illness explanatory models have intensified stigmatising and discriminatory attitudes (Pilgrim and Rogers, 2005). Research has also shown that biogenetic explanations of mental illness are associated with perceptions of dangerousness, unpredictability, and a desire for social distance from people with such diagnoses (Read et al, 2006). Accounts of some participants also reflected such attitudes, arising from staff's mobilisation of illness models of mental distress. For example, Mutya spoke about the judgements made by social services staff about whether she should work or study, and if she was capable of having a romantic relationship due to her diagnosis of borderline personality disorder (BPD), and the personality disorder diagnosis of her partner:

> Social services told me not to get a job and not to go to sixth form. And as I said, education is very important for me. And they were like, basically, 'we think it's going to give you a mental health breakdown if you go sixth form'. But I was like 'why?' Like, this will stop a mental health breakdown, right, to be busy and active within society makes you feel like you have more of a place and more worth, more value. So, I was like, fuck it, I'm going to get a job. And they're like, 'you're not going to be able to keep down a job'. I fucking kept the same job for like six years essentially ... [Relationship with partner is] a very healthy relationship. If it wasn't healthy, then we wouldn't be together, or we wouldn't have even survived this long. Lot of people, my social worker was like, 'it's not going to work because people with BPD can't love', and stuff like that ... She basically thought we were going to make a suicide pact or something [laughs]. Like, she literally said that. She was like 'are you doing this because you are going to try and both commit suicide?' (Mutya, 22 years old, female, Mixed White and Black African)

Participants also talked about feeling as though decisions were made about their mental illness, in terms of diagnosis and treatment, based on their family history of mental illness. Psychiatrists' explanations of, and assumptions about, severe mental illness were imbued with genetic determinism (Bennett et al, 2008), which was often at odds with patients' own understandings of why they had become ill:

> When I was in the hospital, it just felt like I was actually being bullied more than anything. The psychiatrist … had decided that because my Mum had mental health issues and was schizophrenic, and because my brother was schizophrenic, that they needed to treat me along those lines, despite the fact that I'm an individual, I don't drink alcohol, I don't take drugs … It felt like I was being treated by, via stigma because if you've decided that, 'oh your Mum's mentally ill, your brother's got mental illness so you must have some kind of schizophrenia or schizophrenic psychosis as well', I think that's wrong. (Rita, 41 years old, female, Black Caribbean)

Disentangling stigma and racism: 'would he say that to me if I was white?'

The basis of discrimination that participants faced from staff working in mental health services was sometimes difficult to ascertain by participants. Being stigmatised on multiple grounds (Turan et al, 2019) is a common phenomenon, but is often difficult to make sense of, for both the people experiencing multiple or intersecting stigma, and academics who study it. Participants were angry at the poor treatment that they had received from mental health services but were simultaneously perplexed as to whether they were discriminated on the grounds of 'race', their mental illness, or both. Stuart talked in his interview about his concerns at being overmedicated and being told not to work. His thought processes around how this 'might' be due to his 'race' are evident, but he was still uncertain that he was a victim of racism:

> When I'd say, 'am I being discriminated against by the services?', I don't know because I don't know whether there's a conspiracy against me, but it would make a lot of sense … I don't think a doctor's [going to] say 'because you're Black or because you're of African origin, I'm [going to] give you extra medication'. But it's possible like, for example, my current doctor is telling me that I shouldn't work but I'm not [going to] listen to him. But I see that is sort of a form of discrimination, you know, why isn't he taking time and care and saying 'you know what? It's better he works under some sort of regulated, you know, care than me saying he can't work at the moment [because] there's a family'. Would he say that to me if I was white? He might, maybe he would say the same if I was white but, you know, you wouldn't

be doing this research if there wasn't a problem. So, there must be a problem somewhere. (Stuart, 27 years old, male, Mixed White and Black African)

Jasmine recounted the litany of discriminatory experiences with mental health services and social services staff, which she thought were due to having a diagnosis of personality disorder and due to racism. However, like Stuart, she could not pinpoint the exact reason behind the abuse that she had suffered. The stigmatising actions of services (being branded as a liar and attention-seeker, being refused services), along with blatant racist treatment (staff commenting on her skin colour), had ultimately left Jasmine despondent about her future:

> But the thing is, it's very hard to separate out racism, discrimination, and victimisation. There is nobody who looks at things like victimisation. They always assume it must be their interpretation of things. And this kind of universal sort of thing of thinking of mental health, any sort of mental healthcare is good and that people are ultimately there to help. And I think people, researchers, have no idea just how bad and toxic these services are, and how little they don't know anything about people. But they see, about their backgrounds, their history, there's no consideration of trauma people have experienced, that just doesn't come into it. It is ignored. They don't listen to your testimony whatsoever. They treat you as a liar and they dismiss, and negate, everything that you tell them … And nobody will listen to you. I mean, they have written my life off. My life is just a shell, with no prospect of anything. I'm just waiting to die now of, you know, whatever. I'm already dead, you know, that's it. (Jasmine, 50 years old, female, Mixed White and Pakistani)

However, in some participant accounts, experiences of racism, both institutional racism and interpersonal racism, in mental health services were clear to see. There were examples of psychologists and psychiatrists making racist remarks to participants, and sometimes to other patients on hospital wards (interpersonal racism). Rehan recounted being referred to Prevent, the UK's counter-terrorism programme, based on his appearance, because his 'beard got too long'. His account reveals the presence of Islamophobia in the treatment room (institutional racism), and the increasing surveillance role of statutory institutions that provide health and care services (Younis and Jadhav, 2020):

> And, whilst I was going through therapy, one of my counsellors misinterpreted the way … [because] first thing, when you depress[ed] … your grooming goes, you're not bothered how you look, or because

you're slow feeling. And she decided to … refer me to the Prevent team, so that Prevent is the anti-terrorism, right? And luckily for myself, the person that turned up for my house was a person I did the training with. So, it was a totally different conversation. So, we had a cup of tea, we had a laugh, and he left … So that kind of annoyed the social workers, and my psychologist, because nothing came out of that. And then, what I found even more patronising and degrading was, all of a sudden, after about eight or nine sessions, she [counsellor/psychologist] felt threatened by me, whereby you know, like, she had to leave the blinds open, et cetera, et cetera. I'm thinking [pause] what's all this about? (Rehan, 45 years old, male, British Kashmiri)

Participants were racialised (Kapadia and Bradby, 2021) in the therapy room and on hospital wards; stereotypes about how they should behave and feel, and assumptions about their background, were evident in participant narratives. Pauline recounted the racial stereotyping that she was subjected to while staying on a psychiatric ward, and Marcia talked about the racist assumptions of her therapist, thereby showing how racist assumptions and stereotypes about ethnic minority people (interpersonal racism) were providing the basis of how psychologists and psychiatrists treated patients (institutional racism). Consider the following exchange between the interviewer and Pauline (48 years old, female, Black Jamaican):

P: And then one doctor said to me, 'you're a Jamaican. I have a Jamaican friend and he always smiles, and you should be smiling too' … And he was a doctor, a psychiatric doctor … He associated himself with a lot of Jamaican people and they're always bubbling and smiling. Being I'm the only Black person being there at the hospital, he couldn't understand how I could be down one minute and up the next. He thought I should be continuously happy and bubbly and smiley.
Interviewer: Do you remember any more details of that particular moment?
P: I felt low, and I felt disgusted with him, yeah, disgusted with him and I didn't talk to him after that. I didn't bother with him after that. I asked if I could see another psychiatrist.

Likewise, Marcia (47 years old, female, Black Caribbean) said:

Sometimes you'd be sat in a therapy session and, you know, the therapist who's white would say something like, 'oh do you think your problems are, you know, because you come from a poor background?' And I remember thinking, woman, you don't know the first thing about me. Why would you assume that, because I'm Black, I have problems because I come from a poor background?

Conclusion

Our study shows that stigma narratives outside of the prevailing dominant narratives of ethnic minority people's experiences of stigma exist. It must be acknowledged that the Synergi project did not specifically ask participants about stigma. Therefore, there are undoubtedly elements of ethnic minority people's stigma experiences that have not been captured in the data. Nevertheless, our study shows that the structural stigma experienced by ethnic minority people in spaces governed by State institutions cannot be ignored and must form part of the conversations, discourses, and future directions of theorising stigma in these groups. Further, experiences of racism and racialisation cannot be separated easily from stigmatising experiences, and hence it does not make sense to study these separately in future studies, nor should they be conceptualised as operating distinctly from each other in institutional settings such as psychiatric hospitals. Rather, we must move to acknowledging (and operationalising) stigma and racism as two intertwined systems of power (Bonilla-Silva, 1997; Link and Phelan, 2014) that pervade the working practices of mental health services and social services. Shifting the focus (from individual encounters to institutional practices) of where, and how, racial inequalities in mental health services are produced is necessary to begin the process of eradicating inequalities caused by institutional racism and structural stigma.

Could things be different?

- Stigma and racism need to be understood together. Racism and stigma are not usually thought of together. Either people think racism is the cause of poor mental healthcare or they think stigma is. We could substantially improve our understanding of why so many ethnic minority people experience poor mental healthcare treatment if we thought of stigma and racism as operating together and studying them in tandem. This is fundamental to better understanding the problem of ethnic inequalities in mental healthcare.
- More research on mental health professionals' stigmatising views is needed. Research on ethnic minority people and mental illness stigma has tended to focus on the stigmatising views and attitudes of ethnic minority people themselves. Rarely has enough attention been paid to the stigmatising attitudes of mental

healthcare professionals, because people often assume that mental healthcare professionals would not hold stigmatising views about people with mental illness. But this is not the case. We need more research that aims to examine and understand stigmatising attitudes and behaviours of mental health professionals. This would lead to better understandings of why ethnic minority people have poor experiences of mental healthcare, and ultimately inform how their treatment could be improved upon.

- Radical changes to the NHS are needed. There is mental illness stigma among mental health professionals working in the NHS, and there is also evidence of interpersonal and institutional racism being enacted in mental healthcare settings (both inpatient and outpatient). As such, there needs to be an acknowledgement of this and a thorough interrogation of NHS mental healthcare policies and practices to highlight and understand how they systematically disadvantage ethnic minority people and people with severe mental illness. A reform of these policies and practices must be undertaken to remove these disadvantages and produce policies that are grounded within an anti-racist framework. Maybe, then, things really could be different (and better) for ethnic minority people with severe mental illness.

Acknowledgements

This work was funded by the Lankelly Chase Foundation and supported by funding from the Economic and Social Research Council (ESRC) for the Centre on Dynamics of Ethnicity (CoDE) (grant number ES/W000849/1). We would like to acknowledge the invaluable contributions of the co-researchers in the Synergi Collaborative Centre project: Jennifer Edant, Jason Grant-Rowles, Charlotte Maxwell, Zahra Motala, and Sonja Osahan.

References

Bennett, L., Thirlaway, K. and Murray, A.J. (2008) 'The stigmatising implications of presenting schizophrenia as a genetic disease', *Journal of Genetic Counseling*, 17(6): 550–9.

Bonilla-Silva, E. (1997) 'Rethinking racism: toward a structural interpretation', *American Sociological Review*, 62(3): 465–80.

Bonnington, O. and Rose, D. (2014) 'Exploring stigmatisation among people diagnosed with either bipolar disorder or borderline personality disorder: A critical realist analysis', *Social Science and Medicine*, 123: 7–17.

Braun, V. and Clarke, V. (2021) 'One size fits all? What counts as quality practice in (reflexive) thematic analysis?', *Qualitative Research in Psychology*, 18(3): 328–52.

Campbell, R.D. and Mowbray, O. (2016) 'The stigma of depression: Black American experiences', *Journal of Ethnic and Cultural Diversity in Social Work*, 25(4): 253–69.

Corrigan, P.W., Druss, B.G. and Perlick, D.A. (2014) 'The impact of mental illness stigma on seeking and participating in mental health care', *Psychological Science in the Public Interest*, 15(2): 37–70.

Das-Munshi, J., Bhugra, D. and Crawford, M.J. (2018) 'Ethnic minority inequalities in access to treatments for schizophrenia and schizoaffective disorders: Findings from a nationally representative cross-sectional study', *BMC Medical Research Methodology*, 16(55): 1–10.

Department of Health and Social Care (2021) *Reforming the Mental Health Act (White Paper)*, Crown Copyright.

Eylem, O., de Wit, L., van Straten, A., Steubl, L., Melissourgaki, Z., Danışman, G.P. et al (2020) 'Stigma for common mental disorders in racial minorities and majorities: A systematic review and meta-analysis', *BMC Public Health*, 20(1): 1–20.

Fernando, S. (2017) *Institutional Racism in Psychiatry and Clinical Psychology: Race Matters in Mental Health*, Cham: Palgrave Macmillan.

Gary, F.A. (2005) 'Stigma: Barrier to mental health care among ethnic minorities', *Issues in Mental Health Nursing*, 26(10): 979–99.

Gaventa, J. and Cornwall, A. (2008) 'Power and knowledge', in P. Reason and H. Bradbury (eds), *The Sage Handbook of Action Research: Participative Inquiry and Practice* (2nd edn), London: SAGE Publications, pp 172–89.

Goffman, E. (1963) *Stigma: Notes on the Management of Spoiled Identity*, London: Penguin Books Ltd.

Haarmans, M., Nazroo, J., Kapadia, D., Maxwell, C., Osahan, S., Edant, J. et al (2022) 'The practice of participatory action research: Complicity, power and prestige in dialogue with the "racialised mad"', *Sociology of Health and Illness*, 44(S1): 106–23.

Halvorsrud, K., Nazroo, J., Otis, M., Brown Hajdukova, E. and Bhui, K. (2018) 'Ethnic inequalities and pathways to care in psychosis in England: A systematic review and meta-analysis', *BMC Medicine*, 16(1): 1–17.

Hatzenbuehler, M.L. (2016) 'Structural stigma and health inequalities: Research evidence and implications for psychological science', *American Psychologist*, 71(8): 742–51.

Kapadia, D. (2023) 'Stigma, mental illness and ethnicity: Time to centre racism and structural stigma', *Sociology of Health and Illness*, 45: 855–71.

Kapadia, D. and Bradby, H. (2021) 'Ethnicity and health', in C. Chamberlain and A. Lyons (eds) *Routledge International Handbook of Critical Issues in Health and Illness*, London: Routledge, pp 183–96.

Kapadia, D., Zhang, J., Salway, S., Nazroo, J., Booth, A., Villarroel-Williams, N. et al (2022) *Ethnic Inequalities in Healthcare: A Rapid Review*, London: NHS Race and Health Observatory.

Keating, F. (2002) *Breaking the Circles of Fear: A Review of the Relationship Between Mental Health Services and African and Caribbean Communities*, London: Sainsbury Centre for Mental Health.

Link, B.G. and Phelan, J. (2014) 'Stigma power', *Social Science and Medicine*, 103: 24–32.

Macpherson, W. (1999) *The Stephen Lawrence Inquiry. Report of an Inquiry by Sir William Macpherson of Cluny. Cm 4262-I*, London: The Stationery Office.

Memon, A., Taylor, K., Mohebati, L.M., Sundin, J., Cooper, M., Scanlon, T. and de Visser, R. (2016) 'Perceived barriers to accessing mental health services among black and minority ethnic (BME) communities: A qualitative study in Southeast England', *BMJ Open*, 6(11): 1–9.

Misra, S., Jackson, V.W., Chong, J., Choe, K., Tay, C., Wong, J. and Yang, L.H. (2021) 'Systematic review of cultural aspects of stigma and mental illness among racial and ethnic minority groups in the United States: Implications for interventions', *American Journal of Community Psychology*, 68(3–4): 486–512.

Nazroo, J., Bhui, K.S. and Rhodes, J. (2020) 'Where next for understanding race/ethnic inequalities in severe mental illness? Structural, interpersonal and institutional racism', *Sociology of Health and Illness*, 42(2): 262–76.

Pescosolido, B.A. and Martin, J.K. (2015) 'The stigma complex', *Annual Review of Sociology*, 41: 87–116.

Pilgrim, D. and Rogers, A.E. (2005) 'Psychiatrists as social engineers: A study of an anti-stigma campaign', *Social Science and Medicine*, 61: 2546–56.

Read, J., Haslam, N., Sayce, L. and Davies, E. (2006) 'Prejudice and schizophrenia: A review of the "mental illness is an illness like any other" approach', *Acta Psychiatrica Scandinavica*, 114(5): 303–18.

Sheehan, L., Nieweglowski, K. and Corrigan, P. (2016) 'The stigma of personality disorders', *Current Psychiatry Reports*, 18(1): 1–7.

Shefer, G., Rose, D., Nellums, L., Thornicroft, G., Henderson, C. and Evans-Lacko, S. (2013) '"Our community is the worst": The influence of cultural beliefs on stigma, relationships with family and help-seeking in three ethnic communities in London', *The International Journal of Social Psychiatry*, 59(6): 535–44.

Taylor, D. and Richards, D. (2019) 'Triple jeopardy: Complexities of racism, sexism, and ageism on the experiences of mental health stigma among young Canadian Black women of Caribbean descent', *Frontiers in Sociology*, 4: 1–10.

Thornicroft, G., Sunkel, C., Aliev, A.A., Baker, S., Brohan, E., el Chammay, R. et al (2022) 'The Lancet Commission on ending stigma and discrimination in mental health', *The Lancet*, 400(10361): 1438–80.

Trevillion, K., Stuart, R., Ocloo, J., Broeckelmann, E., Jeffreys, S., Jeynes, T. et al (2022) 'Service user perspectives of community mental health services for people with complex emotional needs: A co-produced qualitative interview study', *BMC Psychiatry*, 22(1): 1–18.

Turan, J.M., Elafros, M.A., Logie, C.H., Banik, S., Turan, B., Crockett, K.B. et al (2019) 'Challenges and opportunities in examining and addressing intersectional stigma and health', *BMC Medicine*, 17: 7.

Tyler, I. and Slater, T. (2018) 'Rethinking the sociology of stigma', *The Sociological Review*, 66(4): 721–43.

Wengraf, T. (2001) *Qualitative Research Interviewing*, London: Sage Publications Ltd.

World Psychiatric Association (2019) 'World Psychiatric Association section on stigma and mental illness', *World Psychiatric Association*, [online], Available from: https://3ba346de-fde6-473f-b1da-536498661f9c.filesusr.com/ugd/e172f3_daa6b9755fbc48ecaed4542361c3de72.pdf [Accessed 2 August 2018].

Younis, T. and Jadhav, S. (2020) 'Islamophobia in the National Health Service: An ethnography of institutional racism in PREVENT's counter-radicalisation policy', *Sociology of Health and Illness*, 42(3): 610–26.

2

Stigma and Sexual Arousal: Rethinking HIV-Related Stigma in the Age of PrEP and the Internet

Jaime García-Iglesias

Introduction

The Joint United Nations Programme on HIV/AIDS (UNAIDS, 2018) reaffirms in a 2018 report that HIV-related stigma – meaning 'irrational or negative attitudes, behaviours and judgments driven by fear' – is a key barrier to the fight against HIV worldwide. Stigma hinders HIV prevention, testing, and treatment, and negatively impacts the wellbeing of those already living with HIV who face discrimination in, for example, employment, travel, and healthcare. Most frequently, people experience HIV-related stigma compounded with other sources of stigma, such as homophobia, perceived promiscuity, drug use, poverty, and/or racism. This compounding can be traced back to the early days of the HIV crisis (commencing in 1981), when HIV related stigma was built on a powerful undercurrent of pre-existing homophobia, racism, and moral panics about sex. As Watney (1997, 3) explains, '[f]rom very early on in the history of the epidemic, AIDS has been mobilized to a prior agenda of issues concerning the kind of society we wish to inhabit. These include most of the shibboleths of contemporary "familial" politics, including anti-abortion and anti-gay positions'.

Today when, at least in the Global North, HIV is presented as a chronic manageable condition, stigma remains a key barrier to HIV prevention and treatment efforts, such as the rollout of PrEP (pre-exposure prophylaxis), a HIV prevention drug regime (Witzel et al, 2019). It also continues to negatively impact the lives of both those living with HIV and those perceived to be at risk of contracting the virus, so much so, in fact, that it is a central tenet of much governmental action around HIV (UNAIDS, 2018). As such, it may be surprising to hear Clive, a 49-year-old hotel worker from Essex (UK), saying:

> Nothing turns me on more than fucking with a guy with AIDS. Like, when they're super thin … can barely stand … I [want to] be like that one day. I want people to know how much of a fucking slut I am. And if I die, I'm not too concerned, I'll go happily getting fucked one last time.

Or it may be confusing hearing from Scott, a 53-year-old man living in Australia, who explains: 'I've told doctors I crave HIV in my blood. They were shocked. I think the nurse was kind of … disgusted maybe. They kept asking me why and offering me PrEP. I was turned on to see them like that, thinking I was so twisted.'

Clive and Scott are 'bugchasers', a heterogenous group of gay men who eroticise HIV – a practice known as bugchasing. The term bugchaser encompasses many approaches and attitudes. Some simply fantasise about contracting the virus while enacting measures to prevent actual infection, while others go *all out* in their search for HIV and only stop when they contract it. Some limit their bugchasing to talking in online forums, while others seek to find willing partners offline. Bugchasers are an inroad to exploring how HIV-related stigma is mobilised today. Transcending the initial shock that their comments may trigger allows us to see how their desires and practices complicate existing meanings of HIV-related stigma and require re-evaluating stigma theories and frameworks. After all, as Weeks (1985, 178) writes, 'struggles around sexuality are … struggles over meanings … [S]ex and sexuality are social phenomena shaped in a particular history'. In this way, bugchasers, HIV, and the HIV-stigma they seem to eroticise exist not in isolation, but at the intersection of social, cultural, biomedical, and political moments.

This chapter asks: what role does HIV-related stigma play in bugchasers' sexual lives? What does stigma mean for them? What can bugchasing tell us about stigma? How can we theorise it? How can bugchasing reveal insights about its context, most notably about the contemporary realities of HIV? To do so, this chapter, first, provides an overview of some existing thinking about HIV-related stigma, stigma more generally, and sex. I place emphasis on the work of Plummer (1975) and Parker and Aggleton (2003), but also in the writings of Weeks (1985) and Webster (1984). Doing this allows me to emphasise stigma as interactional and contextual, just as responses to sex (and sex itself) are historical and political. Then, I explore how bugchasers navigate their feelings about stigma. Finally, I discuss how bugchasers' mentions of PrEP and the internet allow us to understand the functioning of these technologies in HIV-related stigma and, more broadly, to better understand HIV today. Thus, I conclude with a reflection on Grov et al's (2014) piece, which argues that we ought to look beyond disease in terms of HIV, to also acknowledge related pleasures and desires. I contend that stigma also requires this rethinking.

HIV and stigma: some thinking

Even the most cursory of searches for HIV and stigma will return an almost endless list of results. Stigma has been identified as a key barrier to HIV prevention (Kippax and Stephenson, 2012; Spieldenner, 2016), treatment and treatment adherence (Race, 2009; Spinelli et al, 2019), quality of life for those living with HIV (Golub et al, 2012), and healthcare provision and scientific research (Watson et al, 2019). Even more generally, HIV-related stigma also negatively impacts the lives of those perceived as being 'at risk' of HIV, such as men who have sex with men (Eaton et al, 2015). While it is impossible to discuss at length all the relevant literature, I would like to focus on two texts that are of particular interest to bugchasing.

Robinson (2013, 103) argues, in an enlightening discussion of bugchasing, that the HIV-positive person 'is seen as "The Other". Someone who has HIV becomes constructed as an irrational actor at some point in one's life and is thus abject within a sexual health discourse and its normative gay male uninfected subject.' That is, living with HIV comes to be constructed through health promotion as signifying a particular past moral or behavioural fault that excludes one from the norm. At the same time, however, seeking to prevent HIV may also generate stigma. This becomes most apparent in relation to PrEP. PrEP is an HIV-prevention strategy that uses antiretroviral drugs (also used in the treatment of HIV infection) to protect HIV negative people from infection. The roll-out of this intervention triggered the appearance of a stigma figure, the 'PrEP whore':

> The PrEP whore is a form of slut shaming. It insists that those who use PrEP are somehow taking a prevention shortcut, a copout from the responsible use of condoms … In this framework, gay men using PrEP deserve to be shunned – socially and sexually. The irony of this construction is that gay men living with HIV are usually stigmatized as sluts. Therefore, both health outcomes – the use of PrEP to prevent HIV acquisition and an HIV infection – lead to the label 'whore'. (Spieldenner, 2016, 1691)

Men who have sex with men have been seen as bearing a disproportionate impact of HIV in its early days, and have since remained associated with

HIV in the cultural narrative and, thus, with its stigma. Weeks (1986, 115, emphasis in original) argues that, during the early days of the AIDS crisis, a slippage took place 'between the idea that homosexuals *caused* "the plague" [HIV] (itself without any backing evidence) to the idea that homosexuality itself was a plague'. This *slippage* served to legitimise pre-existing homophobic narratives (as well as racist and other discriminatory standpoints) in the public eye under the guise of 'health'. Therefore, HIV-related stigma cannot be understood in isolation. It remains deeply linked with the myriad other sources of stigma from which it originates and with which it combines. HIV-related stigma is structural and systemic, cultural and political, because responses to HIV are also structural, systemic, cultural, and political. Crimp (1988, 3) explains:

> HIV does not exist apart from the practices that conceptualise it, represent it, and respond to it. We know AIDS only in and through those practices. This assertion does not contest the existence of viruses, antibodies, infections or transmission routes. Least of all does it contest the reality of illness, suffering, and death. What it does contest is the notion that there is an underlying reality of AIDS.

Crimp, then, describes how the meanings associated with HIV (from stigma to arousal) can only be understood as socially constructed. This requires conceptualising HIV-related stigma (and, in turn, bugchasing arousal) as 'a constantly changing (and often resisted) social process' that 'arises ... and takes shape in special contexts of culture and power' (Parker and Aggleton, 2003, 14, 17). Following this, I find Plummer's (1975) theorising of sexual stigma within the interactionist framework most useful. Plummer posits that sexual stigma is a social construct created and perpetuated through interactions between individuals and societies. According to him, sexual stigma is not inherent to individuals or sexual practices, but rather stigma is imposed on those seen as deviating from societal norms and expectations: 'One always has to consider the "deviant" in relationship to those groups and individuals who define it so' (Plummer, 1975, 20). Sexual stigma becomes a tool of social control used to justify discrimination and inequality. A key takeaway from Plummer's work is that stigma is not limited to specific groups or behaviours, but rather is a pervasive and dynamic phenomenon that can affect all individuals and sexual practices. This approach is similar to Rubin's (1999) argument that the sexual acceptability or deviancy of an act is always established by measuring it against societally established abstractions. Plummer's understanding of stigma as interactional sits well with the above descriptions of HIV as being necessarily the product of specific cultural moments.

Therefore, to understand bugchasing – which evidences a resignification of what HIV and HIV-related stigma mean for men – it becomes necessary that we understand its context; 'sex and sexuality are social phenomena shaped in a particular history' (Weeks, 1985, 178). Doing this, however, may not be as easy as it seems. Sexual desires have long been pushed to the margins of research. To that end, Webster (1984, 391) complained that 'the erotic contours of our imagination remain ... buried in layers of propriety or ambivalence'. This is further emphasised in the case of desires perceived to be deviant or taboo, such as bugchasing, which generates added layers of stigmatisation. Nonetheless, there is value in exploring desires. No matter how shocking or abhorrent bugchasing may seem to many, we cannot forget that even those areas of sexuality deemed taboo are 'simultaneously personal, cultural, political, and social' (Webster, 1984, 391) and, thus, important. Work has already addressed the ways in which apparently troubling sexual fantasies or practices, including barebacking (anal sex without condoms), may, in fact, be illuminating of the cultural, historical, and social contexts in which they exist.

But what is bugchasing exactly? This may be a challenging question to answer. In my research, I have defined bugchasing as the eroticising of HIV, and bugchasers as the men who take part in this practice (García-Iglesias, 2022b). The term bugchaser is not a fixed or stable identity, but rather an umbrella term that encompasses a complex and often contradictory variety of affects, experiences, and practices. As explained in the introduction, some men may seek to engage in sexual encounters to contract HIV, while others may simply fantasise online or take measures to prevent infection, such as using condoms or PrEP (García-Iglesias, 2022a). My previous research of the topic has evidenced that bugchasing is a gay practice, eminently white, and varied in age. Bugchasers, whose desires are not only taboo but also infrequent, have found online to be a perfect space to meet likeminded others, exchange information and talk, and build communities (García-Iglesias, 2020). Some key pieces conceptualising bugchasing from a variety of disciplines are those by Dean (2009), Robinson (2013), and Holmes and O'Byrne (2006).

A wide variety of reasons have been given for bugchasing. Some have argued that it may be a reaction to the cultural imposition of 'safe sex', to the development of effective HIV treatments, to the overwhelming anxiety around HIV that some men may feel, or to feelings of powerlessness (Crossley, 2004). Others have suggested that bugchasers may see HIV as a source of community, solidarity, or connection between men living with HIV, a way to attain a sort of subcultural capital within gay communities as 'old timers', or a form of evidencing masculinity through risk-taking (Dawson et al, 2005; Morris and Paasonen, 2014). Some have further considered that bugchasing may be said to evidence a rebellious dislodging of sexuality from epidemiological concerns and, in turn, an association of HIV with connection, masculinity, and empowerment (Reynolds, 2007). It becomes evident that these different factors and motivations for bugchasing speak to specific cultural and historical moments. For example, the advent of PrEP has transformed many bugchasers' practices and how they articulate their desires, as it has allowed men to *go through the motions* of bugchasing without any risk of contracting HIV (García-Iglesias, 2022a). This proves a profound intersection between bugchasing desires and the contexts in which they originate and operate.

There exists a key challenge at the heart of bugchasing. Bugchasing encompasses many things. For some men, their desires are fleeting. For others, they define their sexual identity. Some men refuse condoms or PrEP, while others embrace them to 'play out their desires' without risk. Some see bugchasing as one of their many desires, whereas others define themselves as 'bugchasers'. This variety may be difficult to theorise:

> The eroticising of HIV and its prevention are not mutually exclusive. Bugchasing is varied: some men enjoy the fantasy with little intention of carrying it out in 'real life', others seek to be infected by any means. Most frequently, men move fluidly in between extremes, sometimes being aroused by the thought of [HIV], sometimes seeking to prevent it for fear of the long-term complications. (García-Iglesias, 2021, 119)

The fact that some men 'just' fantasise about bugchasing, while others act upon it, complicates how we think about stigma – as interactional – in this context. Do only the men who have sex with others – and, thus, make their desires known to them – face stigma? Are those for whom bugchasing is a solitary enterprise free from the risk of stigma? The idea of 'self-labelling' is handy here. Using the example of homosexuality, Plummer (1975, 21) explains that a person does not require others to stigmatise them to feel stigma:

> A person who experiences a homosexual feeling does not have to be hounded out of town, sent to prison, or treated by a psychiatrist to come to see himself as a homosexual. He may quite simply 'indicate' to himself, through the 'interpretation' of the given feeling and the accompanying awareness of the societal hostility, that he is a homosexual.

Therefore, some of the bugchasers whose stories are collected in this chapter simply fantasise about contracting HIV while others actively seek infection by having sex with others and making their desires known. However, both groups (and all the men who sit in between) experience stigma.

The bugchaser stories in this chapter come from a project I conducted between 2018 and 2020, which sought to explore bugchasers' experiences of their own desires, and their use of the internet and of HIV-prevention interventions. More information can be found in my book, *The Eroticizing of HIV* (García-Iglesias, 2022b). As part of the project, I conducted online interviews with 21 men with bugchasing desires. They ranged in age from 25 to 69 years old, and lived in the UK, US, Mexico, Canada, France, Germany, and Australia. The interviews, and the project, sought to understand what bugchasing was, how men experienced it, and how it intersected with the internet and PrEP. What prompted me to write this chapter was that, in their interviews, most men used the term stigma unprompted and in very different ways. While other authors have already discussed the role of stigma in bugchasing, this chapter, rather, seeks to depart from bugchasers' use of the term to understand and theorise its meaning for them.

This chapter considers the role that stigma plays in these men's accounts and problematises the dominant notion of HIV-related stigma by exploring how these men resignify it as arousing. This is an area about which I had been thinking for a long time, since I found it surprising that so many of the participants used the term stigma when talking about their experiences. This, to me, suggested that stigma might be a relevant element to their practices.

Negative experiences of stigma: stigma as shame

Stigma is present in many of the participants' stories. Earlier in this chapter, we read Scott's story about how he was aroused at a nurse being disgusted by his desires. His experience, however, is somewhat of an outlier. Most participants would not share their desires with others (sexual partners, relatives, healthcare providers, and so on). Thus, the stigma they experience is internalised; they 'self-identify' as bugchasers and, using Plummer's (1975) terminology, 'self-react' to the stigma such self-labelling may generate. Dan, a 35-year-old man living in Leeds, explains: 'I keep going through this kind of internal thought process of "what the fuck are you doing?" – excuse my French – "what? Why? What's wrong with you?" I guess there is a set of built-in stigma … or shame … about wanting to do it [bugchasing]. But it's hot.'

Dan has never told anyone about his bugchasing desires, nor has he ever had sex with the intent of contracting the virus (in fact, he said he 'religiously' uses condoms). His bugchasing engagements are limited to talking about it online on a forum under a pseudonym. Thus, he has never been chastised by others (such as relatives and partners), and yet he explicitly describes how stigma compels him to continually question his bugchasing desires and his own worth by assuming that there must be a fault in his character causing his arousal, while also acknowledging that bugchasing 'is hot'. In a similar vein, Giovanni, a 41-year-old man in Canada, tells me: 'I'm not a stupid person, I'm very intelligent, but I have desires that I don't understand. Everybody has their own fantasies and fetishes at different levels, obviously, but this one [bugchasing] I believe is one of the hottest but worse ones.' Like Dan, Giovanni has never talked to anybody about his desires, so his labelling of his desires as 'the worse ones' is self-initiated. What the stories of Dan and Giovanni reveal is that these men engage in a delicate balancing act between stigma being a source of arousal and it simultaneously leading to concern and shame. Even those who, like Giovanni, suggest that bugchasing is 'one of the hottest' desires are also aware of the negative implications that stigma would cause should their desires and/or practices be made public. I ask Giovanni how he would feel if his online bugchasing activity was made public and he answers: 'I would feel exposed, violated. I would feel angry, furious. My safety net, my normal self, would be broken.'

Giovanni's fears resonate with research on HIV and HIV-related stigma that suggests a positive diagnosis leads to a sense of disruption and potential loss of support networks. He suggests that his 'safety net' of peers or friends might ostracise him because of stigma. David, a 28-year-old man living in London, has similar concerns, but reveals some more ambivalence. He has an active Twitter account where he posts videos of himself having sex with men in an attempt to contract HIV. However, he is careful not to show his face: 'Having my face revealed ... I'd absolutely hate that just in case it fell into my work environment. I've got a fairly secure, decent job, and I wouldn't want anything to put that job in jeopardy, not my sex, not me getting the virus.' And yet, a few moments later, he says: 'You see online these men who say they're quitting their jobs, telling everyone, and going to Thailand or somewhere to get it [HIV]. And all that's hot in the moment, to think you could ... like to do all that and not care what people say.'

There is, in David's story, an ambivalence between his concern for the negative and arousing implications of HIV-related and bugchasing-related stigma. In some cases, when bugchasers do share their desires with others, their experiences are equally ambivalent. Brodie, a 33-year-old man from Washington State, US, explained how his previous boyfriend terminated their relationship when Brody shared his bugchasing desires:

> The ex-boyfriend was very negative and left. He was concerned; concerned about me telling him the truth and about all the things like infection and all. I don't know why but I also felt good to be able to do it ... without having to think about ... without worry.

These men mobilise stigma in negative terms, almost as akin to shame; stigma leads to questioning themselves and their desires, to fears about losing their jobs or the disruption of relationships. In this way, stigma elicits similar emotions as those frequently narrated when talking about HIV (such as fear and anxiety). But, at the same time, we also start to see how these men see in stigma a source of arousal – that is, how being 'caught' or 'not caring what people think' are 'hot'. Bugchasing is a unique practice that can complicate and develop the field of stigma research in relation to HIV.

Stigma as arousal

Alongside the acknowledgement of fear and shame, participants (sometimes the same participants) also often speak of stigma as a source of arousal – in some cases as a main source of it. These men are engaging in what Hammond et al (2016) describe as the resignification of the interpretative repertoires of HIV, meaning that they are appropriating existing narratives that surround HIV (such as shame, anxiety, or fear) and developing alternative affective relations to them. For example, Anacleto, a 25-year-old man from Texas (US) who has grown up in a Catholic family of Mexican descent, explains what attracted him to bugchasing initially was not sexual pleasure but, rather, the stigma itself:

> I'd say the stigma, the taboo. That was the first thing. Having sex that was frowned upon, the idea that you're willing to infect yourself with a virus that is sexually transmitted and that it means you don't care of yourself. And then … there came some people out of nowhere that … they embraced it [HIV] and wanted to have it and they wanted to create friendships and relationships based on that.

Anacleto is one of the most committed bugchasers in the sample and had, in fact, been diagnosed with HIV several months before the interview. He is clear: it was the 'stigma' and 'taboo' that drove him to bugchasing. It was not that bugchasing generated additional physical pleasure or that a particular partner was especially attractive, but rather that bugchasing was 'frowned upon'. It was arousing that other men also engaged in it and were chastised for it. He even goes as far as to suggest that it is HIV-related stigma (the association of living with HIV with the idea that a person does not take care of themselves) that he sees as arousing. He explains how verbalised stigma operates as a source of arousal in sexual encounters:

> Oh, yeah, I've had sex where I've told people what I wanted, 'I want you to poz me, I want your toxic load, I want your dirty HIV strain'. And then … yeah … it's arousing to hear that, to hear them tell you how much of a filthy pervert you are.

In the sexual encounter, the verbalisation of HIV-related stigma ('toxic', 'dirty', 'filthy pervert') becomes a source of arousal for Anacleto. He is not alone in describing stigma as arousing in this manner. Gallo, a 38-year-old man from the US, explains that, for him, stigma is arousing, and that pornography is particularly 'hot' when bugchasing is explicit:

> It's the kind of pearl-clutching, the fear, the taboo, the stigma aspect, that is driving me ... In some movies, there are lines where they actually say it ... that they're [going to] give their toxic load or 'do you want my dirty poz load?', and they're saying 'yeah' or begging for it, and there are entire films dedicated to this. So, yeah, it's hot.

Like Anacleto, Gallo finds the stigmatised aspect of bugchasing (the 'pearl-clutching') and the HIV-related stigma ('toxic', 'dirty') arousing (and even inspirational). Anacleto and Gallo seem to wholeheartedly embrace the resignification of HIV and bugchasing related stigma from fear and shame to arousal and pleasure. Most participants, however, are somewhat more ambivalent and engage in a constant negotiation between arousing and negative emotions in terms of their bugchasing. One such example may be Luke, a 28-year-old man from London (UK), who seems conflicted but for whom, nonetheless, bugchasing remains eminently pleasurable:

> I think for me ... it's almost, how can I say it? It's almost like the last taboo ... like the last barrier, because it's so extreme end of the fetish, so shocking, so disgusting for people. I suppose it's maybe that more than the actual infection, the transmission itself, that's why some people take PrEP. I won't lie, it's something that I like, and it does turn me on when I'm thinking about ... it's the fact that you're doing something that's not okay.

Luke confirms the arousing potential of stigma ('the last taboo', 'so disgusting', 'the fact that you're doing something that's not okay') and explains how some people navigate it through PrEP. In this chapter, I have already mentioned PrEP (and the internet – such as in the case of Giovanni or David) several times. I now focus on how these two technologies help men navigate their positive and negative emotions about bugchasing.

Navigating desires through PrEP and the internet

Some of the stories we have already seen have evidenced the key role that PrEP and the internet play in bugchasing. For Giovanni and David, the anonymity of the internet provided a space to experiment with their bugchasing desires. Luke suggested that PrEP might be a way to negotiate arousal while delaying actual infection. It is important that we briefly consider these tools because they necessarily locate bugchasing and its stigma in a particular setting and historical moment. After all, PrEP has only been available since 2012, and websites such as Twitter (now called X) and Tumblr – particularly popular among bugchasers – were founded in 2006 and 2007, respectively. From here, I look at some examples of how these technologies influence bugchasers' emotions around stigma.

The internet, as used by many of the participants, promises anonymity, makes it easy to find likeminded partners, and provides an endless supply of pornography. Scott, the 53-year-old man from Australia who was aroused at his nurse's disgust about his desires, explains online social media as:

> A key component of my daily life, certainly for my sexual life. I get the support from people on Twitter who are there to support me with my desires and I can tell you, quite frankly, that I do not have any one like that to speak to about bugchasing, about my sexual activities.

The internet allows him to engage with others and share the arousal of stigma in specific online spaces, such as Twitter. He goes as far as suggesting that it is the *only* space where he can find this kind of support. However, it may not always be like this for everyone. Earlier in this chapter, I cited a quote from Gallo, a 38-year-old man, who explained how pornography that included bugchasing 'dirty talk', such as 'dirty poz loads' or 'toxic loads', was 'hot'. When asked about the internet, however, he had a different perception:

> It started in my teenage years, on a website called bugshare.net, which I don't think is around anymore. It was erotica and that sort of stuff, and a message board for people to talk. It was hot at first. I had come to see HIV as inevitable and reading about how it could become intimacy, someone else connecting with you in this way, the fact that a man can get pregnant, was kind of interesting and appealing to me in that way. But, pretty quickly, I realised that it was all bullshit, and it kind of … I realised that it [HIV] wouldn't work like that. I could say I stopped doing it for quite a few years because of it.

For Gallo, unlike for Scott, the internet appears as a motivator to reconsider his own emotions around HIV and, in fact, disengage from bugchasing for a period. Similar dynamics can be seen with PrEP. Milo, a 28-year-old man from France, for example, explained how he uses PrEP to prevent HIV-infection while navigating his desire for HIV:

> I don't know how I feel about it yet. I sometimes get loaded by poz guys and it's very, very hot, but I still have that nagging fear sometimes … I'm actually on PrEP, but not all the time. I think it's a great way to stay HIV negative … As many bugchasers say, it's like training wheels for the moment you decide to go without it.

Milo describes how he is still unsure about his emotions in relation to HIV. At times, he finds the potential risk of being infected 'hot', but also has a 'nagging fear'. In this context, he describes how PrEP allows him to 'stay HIV negative' until he 'decides' what to do. This chapter opened with the idea that both stigma and sexual desires were necessarily contextual, social, and political. Bugchasing does not stand in isolation. The way in which bugchasers resignify HIV-related stigma into something that can be arousing can only be understood in relation to the larger society and broader context of HIV in which these men operate. Therefore, the fact that both PrEP and the internet appear as essential elements for how these men navigate their sexual practices and desires evidence that they are, indeed, essential elements for how broader societies understand sexuality (and HIV). This is a context where the availability of the internet and of PrEP is key. PrEP has 'begun to reshape the sexual landscape in many communities' (Auerbach and Hoppe, 2015, 3), and the transformative role of the internet cannot be overstated (Ferreday, 2009). Understanding how bugchasers navigate stigma requires understanding the contexts in which these men operate, but also serves to illuminate those same contexts.

Conclusion

In this chapter, I have explored the existing framework of stigma as developed by Plummer, as well as the difficulties (but importance) of exploring sexuality and sexual desires, especially when they are seen as deviant. I show how HIV-related stigma, most often portrayed as a negative barrier to wellbeing, is resignified by bugchasers. That is, they take stigma, with the negative emotions it generates, to turn it into the erotic object at the centre of their desires and bugchasing practices. This is a direct testament to Plummer's (1975, 30) premise that 'nothing is sexual but naming makes it so'. These men navigate stigma between its associations with shame or fear (the fear of losing relationships or employment) and, most importantly, pleasure and arousal.

While there is some research about the arousing qualities of taboo or deviancy (Webster, 1984; Robinson, 2013), to date, there have been no critical engagements with how HIV-related stigma may be the source of desire and arousal. In undertaking this study, this chapter responds to the call by Parker and Aggleton (2003, 4) to broaden the field of stigma in terms of HIV:

> Our collective inability to more adequately confront stigmatization, discrimination and denial in relation to HIV and AIDS is linked to the relative theoretical and methodological tools available to us. It is important, therefore, to critically evaluate the available literature on

the study of stigma and discrimination, both independent of HIV/AIDS and more specifically in relation to it, in order to develop a more adequate conceptual framework for thinking about the nature of these processes, for analysing the ways in which they work in relation to HIV and AIDS.

I placed the emphasis of the first section of this chapter on the notion that stigma is interactional and comes to be in social interactions, and how no act or person is intrinsically stigmatised. These bugchasers' accounts push this further to suggest that the meaning of stigma itself also comes to be built through those interactions. This is why this chapter has focused not on imposing extraneous theoretical frameworks on these men's experiences, but rather to explore and theorise them as they are lived in their everyday lives.

Men like Scott or Giovanni suggest we cannot assume that HIV-related stigma will always, or only, lead to negative emotions. Rather, their stories evidence how there is a complex, and sometimes contradictory, navigation of both negative *and* positive or arousing emotions. This resonates with Grov et al's (2014, 403) call for an approach to HIV research that considers not only disease prevention, but also sex itself:

> Many of our research questions remain grounded in models of disease prevention … Yet we can only wonder what other questions might have been explored were we not so focused on preventing HIV … It may be that previous efforts have resulted in a body of literature about gay and bisexual men that is disease-focused and has not fully allowed for an exploration of the manner in which these men construct their sexual lives.

That is, when exploring HIV-related stigma, bugchasers evidence the need to move beyond a limited thinking about disease, prevention, and discrimination, to a more complex approach that also considers pleasure and arousal. I have also argued, at the beginning of this chapter, that sexual desires – even, or perhaps especially, those that are deemed deviant – are closely connected to the social context in which they arise and can be enlightening of their broader political, social, or cultural realities. The important role that PrEP and the internet play in bugchasers' resignification of HIV-related stigma evidences the transformative role that both technologies have had in HIV and sexuality more broadly. Bugchasing, therefore, is not an isolated niche of deviants disconnected from reality. Rather, exploring and explaining their desires and practices also sheds light on the larger shifts and changes that HIV and sexuality have experienced in the last decades.

Could things be different?

- Stigma can, and does, hurt people. It hurts those living with HIV daily. It poses sometimes unsurmountable barriers to them living fulfilling lives. But not everybody reacts to and experiences stigma in the same way. We need to be open to understanding that stigma may also provoke and produce emotions that are not negatively experienced, but rather can be arousing or pleasurable.
- Based on this, policies related to stigma, particularly those that inform and shape health promotion, should acknowledge this complexity while continuing to fight for a world where people living with HIV do not face discrimination or fear.
- In research, disciplines across the board should embrace ambivalence as key to understanding how people can experience stigma differently. It is far more common than many people appreciate that both negative and harmful and positive and pleasurable experiences of stigma coexist in complex or seemingly contradictory ways. Recognising this would support the development of better policy, health promotion, and healthcare.

References

Auerbach, J.D. and Hoppe, T.A. (2015) 'Beyond "getting drugs into bodies": Social science perspectives on pre-exposure prophylaxis for HIV', *Journal of the International AIDS Society*, 18(4 Suppl 3): 19983.

Crimp, D. (ed) (1988) *AIDS: Cultural Analysis/Cultural Activism*, Cambridge, MA: MIT Press.

Crossley, M.L. (2004) 'Making sense of "barebacking": Gay men's narratives, unsafe sex and the "resistance habitus"', *British Journal of Social Psychology*, 43(2): 225–44.

Dawson, A.G., Ross, M.W., Henry, D. and Freeman, A. (2005) 'Evidence of HIV transmission risk in barebacking men-who-have-sex-with-men: Cases from the internet', *Journal of Gay and Lesbian Psychotherapy*, 9(3–4): 73–83.

Dean, T. (2009) *Unlimited Intimacy: Reflections on the Subculture of Barebacking*, Chicago: University of Chicago Press.

Eaton, L.A., Driffin, D.D., Kegler, C., Smith, H., Conway-Washington, C., White, D. and Cherry, C. (2015) 'The role of stigma and medical mistrust in the routine health care engagement of Black men who have sex with men', *American Journal of Public Health*, 105(2): e75–82.

Ferreday, D. (2009) *Online Belongings: Fantasy, Affect and Web Communities*, Oxford: Peter Lang.

García-Iglesias, J. (2020) 'Writing bugchasing ethnoperformance: Creative representations of online interactions', *Sexualities*, 24(1–2): 154–75.

García-Iglesias, J. (2021) 'From training wheels to chemical condoms: Exploring narratives of prep discontinuation', *Health*, 27(1): 114–28.

García-Iglesias, J. (2022a) '"PrEP is like an adult using floaties": Meanings and new identities of prep among a niche sample of gay men' *Culture, Health & Sexuality*, 24(2): 153–66.

García-Iglesias, J. (2022b) *The Eroticizing of HIV: Viral Fantasies*, Cham: Springer International Publishing.

Golub, S.A., Starks, T.J., Payton, G. and Parsons, J.T. (2012) 'The critical role of intimacy in the sexual risk behaviours of gay and bisexual men', *AIDS Behaviour*, 16(3): 626–32.

Grov, C., Breslow, A.S., Newcomb, M.E., Rosenberger, J.G. and Bauermeister, J.A. (2014) 'Gay and bisexual men's use of the internet: Research from the 1990s through 2013', *Journal of Sex Research*, 51(4): 390–409.

Hammond, C., Holmes, D. and Mercier, M. 2016) 'Breeding new forms of life: A critical reflection on extreme variances of bareback sex', *Nursing Inquiry*, 23(3): 267–77.

Holmes, D. and O'Byrne, P. (2006) 'Bareback sex and the law: The difficult issue of HIV status disclosure', *Journal of Psychosocial Nursing and Mental Health Services*, 44(7): 26–33.

Kippax, S. and Stephenson, N. (2012) 'Beyond the distinction between biomedical and social dimensions of HIV prevention through the lens of a social public health', *American Journal of Public Health*, 102(5): 789–99.

Morris, P. and Paasonen, S. (2014) 'Risk and utopia', *GLQ: A Journal of Lesbian and Gay Studies*, 20(3): 215–39.

Parker, R. and Aggleton, P. (2003) 'HIV and AIDS-related stigma and discrimination: A conceptual framework and implications for action', *Social Science and Medicine*, 57(1): 13–24.

Plummer, K. (1975) *Sexual Stigma: An Interactionist Account*, London: Routledge and Kegan Paul.

Race, K. (2009) *Pleasure Consuming Medicine: The Queer Politics of Drugs*, Durham: Duke University Press.

Reynolds, E. (2007) '"Pass the cream, hold the butter": Meanings of HIV positive semen for bugchasers and giftgivers', *Anthropology and Medicine*, 14(3): 259–66.

Robinson, B.A. (2013) 'The queer potentiality of barebacking: Charging, whoring, and breeding as utopian practices', in A. Jones (ed), *A Critical Inquiry into Queer Utopias*, New York: Palgrave Macmillan, pp 101–28.

Rubin, G.S. (1999) *Thinking Sex: Notes for a Radical Theory of the Politics of Sexuality*, New York: Routledge.

Spieldenner, A. (2016) 'Prep whores and HIV prevention: The queer communication of HIV pre-exposure prophylaxis (PrEP)', *Journal of Homosexuality*, 63(12): 1685–97.

Spinelli, M.A., Scott, H.M., Vittinghoff, E., Liu, A.Y., Gonzalez, R., Morehead-Gee, A. et al (2019) 'Missed visits associated with future preexposure prophylaxis (PrEP) discontinuation among prep users in a municipal primary care health network', *Open Forum Infectious Diseases*, 6(4): ofz101.

UNAIDS (2018) *Global Partnership for Action to Eliminate All Forms of HIV-Related Stigma and Discrimination*, Geneva: UNAIDS.

Watney, S. (1997) *Policing Desire: Photography, Aids and the Media*, London: Cassell.

Watson, S., Namiba, A. and Lynn, V. (2019) 'NHIVNA best practice. The language of HIV: A guide for nurses', *HIV Nursing*, 19(2): BP1–4.

Webster, P. (1984) 'The forbidden: Eroticism and taboo', in C.S. Vance (ed), *Pleasure and Danger: Exploring Female Sexuality*, Boston: Routledge and Kegan Paul, pp 385–98.

Weeks, J. (1985) *Sexuality and its Discontents: Meanings, Myths, and Modern Sexualities*, London: Routledge.

Weeks, J. (1986) *Sexuality*, New York: Routledge.

Witzel, T.C., Nutland, W. and Bourne, A. (2019) 'What are the motivations and barriers to pre-exposure prophylaxis (PrEP) use among Black men who have sex with men aged 18–45 in London? Results from a qualitative study', *Sexually Transmitted Infections*, 95(4): 262–66.

3

The Contested Nature of Abortion Stigma: From the Individual to the Structural

Gillian Love

Introduction

Abortion – the intentional ending of a pregnancy – is stigmatised in almost all contexts globally (Shellenberg et al, 2011; Cockrill et al, 2013; Purcell et al, 2014; Hanschmidt et al, 2016). Legal frameworks vary widely, from jurisdictions in which abortion is completely illegal (such as El Salvador, Honduras, and Nicaragua) to those in which abortion is completely decriminalised (such as Canada) (Center for Reproductive Rights, 2022). Academic literature has noted that abortion stigma exists even in otherwise liberal contexts (Shellenberg et al, 2011; Cárdenas et al, 2018), meaning that those who have abortions may feel the need to keep their abortions secret (Astbury-Ward et al, 2012), anticipate negative reactions from others (Shellenberg et al, 2011), and internalise negative self-evaluations as a result of ending a pregnancy (Cockrill and Nack, 2013).

The most influential definition of abortion stigma is perhaps that of Kumar et al (2009, 628), who describe it as 'a negative attribute ascribed to women who seek to terminate a pregnancy that marks them, internally or externally, as inferior to ideals of womanhood'. This definition points to the important social and cultural elements of abortion stigma; women are generally expected to be instinctively nurturing, naturally fertile, and inevitably mothers. Ending a pregnancy transgresses each of these feminine ideals (Kumar et al, 2009). Since the publication of Kumar et al's work, discussion and debate has continued about how to define and delineate abortion stigma as a concept (Hessini, 2014), whether it has been misapplied (Kumar, 2013), what theoretical perspectives might be preferrable

(Beynon-Jones, 2017; Millar, 2020), and whether researchers have overstated stigma and ignored more nuanced or positive aspects of abortion (Baird and Millar, 2019; Purcell et al, 2020).

In this chapter, I map some of the more recent developments in conceptualising abortion stigma. The chapter begins with the dominance of psychological and quantitative understandings of abortion stigma, and the tendency in this work to frame abortion stigma as a static attribute that one can possess or impose on to others. The remainder of the chapter offers alternative approaches to conceptualising abortion stigma that understand stigma as an operation of power (Parker and Aggleton, 2003; Tyler, 2020). To do so, I propose a typology of four 'power-attendant' approaches to understanding abortion stigma: the first is discursive; the second, intersectional; the third, biopolitical; and the fourth, embodied. These four approaches complement and overlap one another significantly, as they are scaffolded by a range of complementary theoretical and conceptual frameworks. Their meanings, significance, and relationship to the concept of power will be explained throughout the chapter, but each approach fundamentally understands stigma to be a regulatory function of power, often State-sanctioned, rather than an unfortunate social ill that might be solved by 'raising awareness' (Tyler and Slater, 2018).

While stigma is not *the* defining feature of abortion, it is a significant concept on both a micro- and macro-level. Conceptualising abortion stigma in a manner that is attendant to power and dominance is part of a wider project in the sociology of health and illness (and particularly this book) to revisit stigma as a productive and political concept (Scambler, 2018; Tyler and Slater, 2018). Understanding how abortion stigma is produced and maintained has material consequences globally for individuals, communities, and societies.

Challenging individualised and psychological models of stigma

As with much of the wider literature on stigma, work on abortion stigma has taken many cues from Goffman's (1963, 3) formulation of stigma as an attribute that is 'deeply discrediting' due to its relationship to stereotypes. This literature paints a picture of the experience of abortion stigma which, while not universal or the defining feature of abortion, is nevertheless common. The fear of negative social attitudes and anticipated judgement from others appears to affect women's likelihood of disclosure long after having an abortion (Astbury-Ward et al, 2012; Hanschmidt et al, 2016), and keeping abortion a secret can have negative psychological consequences, such as distressing and intrusive thoughts (Major and Gramzow, 1999).

The fear of being judged (often called 'felt stigma' in the literature) is partly influenced by the mainstream media which, in the UK, depicts abortion as a negative and risky practice associated with other 'discredited' social practices like promiscuity, teenage pregnancy, and rape (Purcell et al, 2014). It is also partly influenced by contextual understandings of the status of abortion as a discredited practice, for example, in conservative and religious contexts (Cárdenas et al, 2018).

Experiencing enacted or anticipated stigma can also be accompanied by 'internalised' stigma, in which those who have abortions internalise negative perceptions about abortion (Shellenberg et al, 2011), and engage in numerous individual stigma management strategies related to self-image and reputation (Cockrill and Nack, 2013). Internalised abortion stigma in these studies manifests as beliefs that women who have abortions (including the participants) are careless and irresponsible, feel guilt, and should be prevented from or punished for having abortions (Cockrill and Nack, 2013). Some manage these thoughts and feelings through 'stigma management strategies', like excusing or justifying their own abortions while denigrating others, a strategy Cockrill and Nack (2013, 982) refer to as 'stigma transference'.

Sociological literature has offered insights into how abortion stigma is produced and sustained. Kimport et al (2011) have argued that, rather than the abortion itself, it is the social and political context of the person who has the abortion that often produces emotional difficulties. Furthermore, they identify a division of labour between women and men regarding pregnancy prevention, abortion, and childrearing. As a result, 'the majority of abortion-related emotional burdens fall on women' (Kimport et al, 2011, 103). Kirkman et al's (2011) discursive analysis of women contemplating abortion also emphasises the importance of the complex personal and social contexts in which stigma is produced, and Hoggart's (2017) work on internalised abortion stigma has explored the way women construct alternative narratives of responsibility and morality in the face of social norms which position abortion as a discrediting attribute. Finally, literature on stigma intervention has detailed efforts to evaluate community-level education and storytelling around abortion, to mixed effect (Bloomer et al, 2017; Belfrage et al, 2020; Cutler et al, 2022).

While this literature offers important insights into the experience and operation of abortion stigma, it has also attracted some criticism. First, approaching stigma as largely a property that individuals carry, or that individuals impose onto others, in ways that are static and quantifiable, has been critiqued for ignoring the structural elements of stigma, and its shifting and situated qualities (Beynon-Jones, 2017; Millar, 2020; Love, 2021). This is particularly evident in the (largely psychological) literature that has approached abortion stigma as something quantifiable and measurable via scales (Cockrill et al, 2013; Sorhaindo et al, 2016; Hanschmidt et al, 2018; Martin et al, 2018; Cetinkaya et al, 2019). Second, it has been noted that in the 'geography' of health stigma (Heijnders and Van Der Meij, 2006), abortion stigma literature tends to concentrate on individual and community levels, neglecting wider levels such as framing discourses and mass culture, governmental/structural levels, and organisational/institutional levels (Kumar et al, 2009).

Abortion stigma scholars have only marginally engaged with sociological theorisations of stigma that foreground power and the 'political economy' of stigma (Parker and Aggleton, 2003). Yet, these approaches offer useful ways into the aforementioned neglected 'levels' of abortion stigma. This strand of stigma scholarship understands stigma as a regulatory function of power, often State-sanctioned, rather than an unfortunate social ill that might be solved by 'raising awareness' (Tyler and Slater, 2018). The production of stigma in this scholarship has been argued to act as an explicit mechanism to denigrate those at the bottom of systems of oppression and marginalisation, thereby shoring up support for punitive State sanctions against them (Parker and Aggleton, 2003; Jones, 2013; Weissman, 2017; Tyler, 2020). Using this definition of stigma as a foundation, in the following sections, I map out my typology of the scholarship that has engaged with abortion stigma on these terms: discursive approaches, intersectional approaches, biopolitical approaches, and embodied approaches.

Discourse and identity

The 'roots' of abortion stigma, it has been argued by Hoggart (2017), are social constructions. These include: narrow gender roles, intent to control female sexuality, and compulsory motherhood (Kumar et al, 2009); attribution of personhood to the foetus (Hopkins et al, 2005); religion; and media discourse (Purcell et al, 2014). One strand of scholarship on abortion seeks to understand these elements as *discursive formations*. Discourse refers to systems of meaning and language that produce concepts, identities, and people. Thinking discursively means thinking about who/what has the power to produce, and who/what is fixed in place by discourse (Foucault, 1998; Skeggs, 2004). Thinking about abortion discursively allows us to move away from 'reifying' stigma and turn our analytical attention to the ongoing, constantly negotiated nature of stigma. This is the thrust of Beynon-Jones' (2017, 227) work on abortion stories, in which stigma is understood to be a 'reproduction of social relations of power which depend on differentiating "normal" from "deviant" identities through discourse'. In approaching interview data from women who have had abortions discursively, rather than thinking of their stories as transparent evidence of something static and stable, Beynon-Jones demonstrates that women often do discursive labour to negotiate non-stigmatised identities, for example, through positioning their abortion decisions as certain or common sense. This discursive approach prompts us to understand stigmatised identities as something that people are actively engaged in negotiating, not something they simply possess.

A discursive approach also prompts us to think about how individual narratives are connected to wider systems of meaning. Abortion discourse politically tends to be understood as a battle between two positions: 1) pro-choice positions that focus on abortion as healthcare, the discourse of bodily autonomy, and present foetuses as inanimate objects or biological matter in order to normalise the procedure (Broussard, 2020; MYA Network, n.d.); and 2) pro-life positions that draw on the discourse of rights to infer personhood onto pregnancies from their earliest stages, evoking disgust and sorrow through images (often doctored) of foetuses, as well as the belief that abortion is harmful and therefore 'anti-women' (Hopkins et al, 2005; Wyatt and Hughes, 2009; Roberti, 2021). Outside of the (somewhat reductive) dichotomy between medicalised pro-choice discourse and emotive anti-abortion positions, other positions are legitimised by political and public discourse around abortion. For example, it is not uncommon for 'moderate' pro-choice positions to carefully cede ground to the understanding of abortion as a negative or harmful phenomenon, while advocating that merciful and just societies must tolerate it. This is the position that some pro-abortion campaigns took up during the Irish abortion referendum as an explicit strategy to appeal to 'Middle Ireland', emphasising individual women's stories and compassion rather than explicit messages around bodily autonomy or choice (Cullen and Korolczuk, 2019).

Embracing a conceptualisation of abortion stigma that focuses on its shifting, discursive elements does not detract from the idea that Kumar et al (2009) usefully point out: stigma often arises from quite fixed ideas about what it means to be pregnant or be a woman. While Kumar et al suggest there are 'universal' ideals of womanhood that shape abortion stigma, they also point out that it can also have a local character, just as Tyler and Slater (2018) identify stigma as a 'local operation of power'. What becomes clear from the narratives of those who have abortions is that people are often engaged actively in these local contestations over the meaning of abortion and pregnancy (Love, 2021).

Approaching abortion stigma discursively can usefully bring together the micro-level, individual contestations of meaning in abortion stories, and the macro-level, political and social frameworks that they exist within. This approach pushes against the conceptualisation of stigma as a stable or measurable attribute that one can possess or impose onto others. Instead, a discursive approach draws attention to the diffuse nature of power.

Intersections of stigma

As well as thinking about power and discourse at the level of identity formation, some have also written about abortion stigma as part of a process of producing social inequality. As Tyler (2020) and Slater (2018) have argued, stigma performs a regulatory function. In considering the regulatory function of abortion stigma, it is productive to begin with gender. Feminist scholars and activists have long established that the regulation of abortion is a proxy for the regulation of women (even if it is also accessed by people of other genders). Women's reproductive freedom and agency has been associated with positive outcomes. Access to abortion is associated with better physical and mental health outcomes than being denied abortion (Biggs et al, 2017; Rocca et al, 2021). Conversely, criminalising abortion does not necessarily decrease its prevalence significantly, leads to dangerous and even fatal outcomes for those seeking abortion, and leads to forced birth (Ahman and Shah, 2011; Faundes and Shah, 2015). Feminists have, therefore, historically positioned abortion as an essential political issue (Petchesky, 1990; Sheldon, 1997; Sanger, 2017).

If we pull back our frame of analysis from abortion, it is also true to say that womanhood is socially, culturally, and biologically associated with motherhood, childbearing, and child-rearing. Thus, when Kumar et al (2009, 628) define abortion stigma as marking women as 'inferior to ideals of womanhood', they are referring to 'universal' feminine ideals that associate women with fecundity, being nurturing, and self-sacrifice. We can trouble this definition by bringing it into conversation with theorisations of stigma as an explicit manufacturing of consent for punitive measures against the most marginalised (Tyler, 2020), beginning with the fact that all women are *not* universally expected or encouraged to reproduce. Kumar et al's (2009) definition of abortion stigma treats gender as a *single axis* of oppression and marginalisation rather than a part of a 'matrix of domination' inflected by race, sexuality, disability, and so on (Hill Collins, 2002). The theoretical framework of intersectionality views domination and oppression as multi-axis issues that constitute one another and is, therefore, a useful framework with which to consider how gender is intertwined with other structures (Crenshaw, 1991).

Women historically prevented from reproduction, rather than being expected to reproduce, include Black and Indigenous women who have been targeted in some nation-states with programmes of sterilisation (Pegoraro, 2015; Vergès, 2018), as well as 'softer' barriers to reproduction including systemic poverty, structural violence, and vilification (Silliman, 2004; Forward Together, 2005). Involuntary sterilisation has also historically affected disabled and mentally ill women in Canada (Amy and Rowlands, 2018) and Sweden (Boréus, 2006). Some jurisdictions require transgender people to be sterilised if they wish to gain legal recognition of their gender (Dunne, 2017; Repo, 2019), and options for preservation of fertility are not always well understood (Nixon, 2013; Chen et al, 2017).

More diffuse and implicit barriers exist for some groups. Young, working-class, poor women's abortion requests are often deemed understandable by many healthcare professionals in the UK, who express an explicit or implicit judgement that these 'types' of women make poor mothers (Skeggs, 1997; Tyler, 2008). In contrast, abortion requests from middle-class, professional women in stable relationships of the 'right' age are more likely to be questioned (Lee et al, 2004; Beynon-Jones, 2013). Furthermore, the 'discursive resources' that middle-class women can access to present their abortions as 'understandable' are often bound up with pressure to conform to ideal neoliberal femininity – that is, of being adaptable, self-regulating, and respectable (Love, 2021).

It is clear, then, that abortion stigma is intimately connected to other forms of reproductive stigma that punish some for reproducing and others for choosing not to. The 'arrangements by which some reproductive futures are valued while others are despised' (Ginsburg and Rapp, 1995, 3) has been called 'stratified reproduction' (Colen, 1995). The term 'repronormativity' has also been used to describe the hegemonic discourse that reproduction is between heterosexual, cisgender couples, and marks reproduction outside of these arrangements as deviant (Karaian, 2013; Weissman, 2017).

Thinking about abortion stigma in terms of structural arrangements is less common in the academic literature, but it is modelled in other ways by community and activist movements. As has been pointed out before (Millar, 2020), the Reproductive Justice movement founded and sustained by Women of Colour in the US engages explicitly with reproductive stigma and inequality as a social and political arrangement that requires individual and community resistance and radical structural change to remedy (Silliman, 2004; Forward Together, 2005; SisterSong Collective, n.d.). Organisations like SisterSong and Forward Together draw attention to the intersections of gender, race, class, and disability that produce conditions whereby communities must fight not only for the right to abortion, but the right to have children and to parent. However, academic work on abortion stigma has yet to meaningfully engage with frameworks like Reproductive Justice to conceptualise abortion stigma.

Without considering stigma intersectionally, these dimensions of reproductive injustice remain invisible in discussions around abortion. While some have argued for strictly delineating between abortion stigma and other types of reproductive stigma (Kumar, 2013; Hessini, 2014), considering them as intertwined manifestations of inequality is useful for two reasons. First, the explicit, State-sanctioned stigmatisation of marginalised groups – the stigma machine (Tyler, 2020) – creates hegemonic consensus around who has a right to reproduce, and who has the right to *opt out* of reproduction, a context essential to understanding abortion stigma. Second, our definitions of stigma risk reifying this hegemonic consensus rather than challenging it.

Biopolitics

Conceptualising stigma as intersectional and as intimately bound with other forms of reproductive stigma allows us to understand local operations of power. On a global level, and on the level of individual nation-states, this approach also allows us to engage with active projects invested in generating and maintaining stigma in order to sustain or produce particular social orders. We might conceive of these projects as *biopolitical*. Biopolitics describes the birth, death, and reproduction of the population facilitated by 'a series of interventions and regulatory controls' that operate on two levels at once, namely, the level of the individual body and the level of the population (Foucault, 1978, 139).

Abortion stigma is bound up with these projects in complex ways. For example, States concerned with falling birth rates and ageing populations might encourage pro-natalist policies; they need babies, and therefore criminalise and stigmatise abortion. Poland offers an example of this kind of pro-natalist project. After the fall of Communism, Poland has seen a decline in birth rate, and the government has imposed restrictions on abortion and contraception (Mishtal, 2012; Cullen and Korolczuk, 2019). Even though the declining birth rate is partly a response to the removal of socialist, motherhood-friendly policies like subsidised childcare, maternity leave, and healthcare, the Polish State has embarked on a project of framing Polish women who do not have children as selfish, encouraging them to have children in the name of economic and nationalist causes (Mishtal, 2012). Conversely, anti-natalist States encourage or enforce abortion and contraception, and stigmatise 'irresponsible' reproduction, to curb what they frame as damaging overpopulation; China's one-child policy era is an example of this (Green, 1988).

In this sense, abortion and abortion stigma can be understood within a broader 'political economy' of stigma in which social inequality is produced to promote particular ends (Parker and Aggleton, 2003). While explicit and 'strong' eugenics is not widely practiced today in most nations, 'weak' forms of eugenics arguably do operate in many contexts in which only non-disabled, middle-class, heterosexual and cisgender people are explicitly encouraged to reproduce (Shakespeare, 1998; Weissman, 2017). In this sense, abortion stigma can be seen as the driver of wider aims.

The relationship between reproduction, abortion, and nationalism offers one window into the workings of biopolitics (Yuval-Davis, 1996). The 2019 abortion referendum in Ireland to repeal or retain the eighth amendment of the constitution, which criminalised abortion in most cases, offers a case study. Irish reproductive politics is heavily implicated with questions of sexual citizenship, nationhood, and religiosity. In particular, the referendum prompted renewed conversation around the relationship between the

Catholic Church and pro-natalism, as well as reckoning with histories of abuse of young women who had babies out of wedlock (Simpson et al, 2014). The campaign to repeal the eighth amendment and legalise abortion focused on constituting Ireland as a country with a past and present of uncaring treatment of women, but focused on the possibilities of embracing care and compassion, and treating women with dignity (Cullen and Korolczuk, 2019; Together For Yes, n.d.). The successful campaign to legalise abortion was characterised by Taoiseach Leo Varadkar as the day Ireland 'threw off the last shadows of the nation's conservative past' (Ó Cionnaith, 2018).

However, the anti-abortion campaign to 'Save the 8th' also focused on constituting Ireland as a compassionate nation. Campaign materials invoked the idea of Ireland as safe and welcoming for pregnant women where 'babies are valued and protected', an Ireland that 'values the best from our history and the promise of our future', contrasted with the British track record of aborting babies with Down's syndrome (Save the 8th, n.d.). The stigmatisation of abortion as a cruel, prejudiced, and uncaring practice that harms women and vulnerable babies is used here in service of a national image of Ireland as a diverse and inclusive nation.

Abortion stigma, and other forms of reproductive stigma, are therefore not incidental or accidental. While it might be true that, on an individual level, people may face abortion stigma because they 'inadvertently challeng[e] widely held assumptions about the "essential nature" of women' (Kumar et al, 2009, 628), stigma on a biopolitical level is not inadvertent, and cannot be solved through interventions aimed at community-level tolerance or education (Parker and Aggleton, 2003).

Embodiment

If abortion stigma can productively be understood as a regulatory mechanism of power, and as biopolitical, another dimension of our thinking must be about how abortion stigma might be embodied. Embodiment, in social theory, refers not simply to the sensations of the body, but the process by which bodies are made material, and how we make sense of their materiality (McNay, 1991; Shilling, 2007). A clear example of how embodiment can be an important element of stigma is Williams and Annandale's (2020, 428) work on weight stigma, which they suggest directly impacts people's 'objective and subjective experiences of their bodies'. In their study of weight-loss groups, participants literally felt heavier after engaging in behaviours associated with weight gain even if the number on the scale remained the same. In this example, the materiality of the body is experienced and interpreted through available discursive formations, constantly shifting and being constructed rather than being a stable, static object. Williams and Annandale point out that scholars of stigma tend to think about the *cognitive* elements of stigma, whereby 'felt' stigma is usually understood to mean anticipation and expectation of poor treatment (Herek, 2009). Their work suggests that the *feeling* of stigma can also be embodied (Williams and Annandale, 2020).

Even though pregnancy and abortion are firmly embodied experiences, literature on abortion stigma has neglected the body, and even social scientific literature on abortion experiences more broadly reflect this absence. However, literature that does approach abortion stigma through the lens of embodiment feature two concepts prominently: the 'natural' and pain.

The concept of the 'natural' is writ large in discourse around pregnancy and childbirth, often contrasted with medicalisation (Johnson, 2008). 'Normal' or 'natural' childbirth was an explicit goal in UK midwifery, for example, for many years. Proponents of 'normal' childbirth aimed to encourage births with as little medical intervention as possible (Maternity Care Working Party, 2007). 'Natural' abortion emerges as a concept in several studies about abortion embodiment, particularly for those who have medical abortions (Purcell et al, 2017; Broussard, 2020; Siegel, 2020; Love, 2021). Abortion is typically administered either medically with a combination of the medicines misoprostol and mifepristone, or surgically through procedures including vacuum aspiration (in early pregnancy) and dilation and curettage. Some people are offered a choice of method, depending on their gestation and the resources of their providers, but many people are only offered one option or encouraged to consider one or the other.

Medical abortions seem to be experiences more closely associated with corporeality, as they require the pregnant person to remain conscious and 'pass' the pregnancy at home or in hospital (Purcell et al, 2017). For those who have medical abortions in the first trimester, medical abortions are typically passed at home and are often compared to a heavy period (Broussard, 2020), whereas medical abortions in the second trimester are usually passed in hospital settings and involve a more physical 'labour' (Purcell et al, 2017). Making sense of this experience as a 'natural' alternative to a surgical procedure is sometimes involved in stigma management, as it can position the speaker as passive, whereas for others, making sense of their abortion as akin to other 'natural' experiences like miscarriage or labour allowed them to position their experiences as normal and untroubled (Siegel, 2020).

The second common concept in literature on abortion and embodiment is that of pain. Making sense of pain and emotional reactions to it are a complex and nuanced part of many people's abortion experiences (Purcell et al, 2017; Broussard, 2020; Love, 2021). For some, the pain involved in medical abortion is experienced as necessary, and a bodily sign that the pregnancy is over; pain 'signifie[s] the arrival of a desired outcome' (Broussard, 2020, 5), and can therefore be a neutral or positive aspect of the experience. However, the internalisation of stigma and shame can lead some to experience pain and discomfort as deserved. For example, in Purcell et al's (2017) study of second trimester medical abortion experiences, some participants felt they didn't 'deserve' pain relief. Broussard (2020) also noted several participants felt the same about their early medical abortions. In my own study, more than one participant expressed the idea that their abortions were something to suffer through in order to gain redemption or prevent future abortions (Love, 2021). These insights demonstrate that stigma can not only be 'felt' in a cognitive sense, but also in an embodied sense.

However, as Kumar (2013) reminds us, a focus on stigma can assign it too much importance and hinder us from seeing sites of resistance to, or absence of, stigma. Resistance to embodied stigma was a feature of some participants' stories in my own study of abortion narratives in England (Love, 2021). One participant described the transformative affect her abortion had on her relationship with her body, as it forced an understanding of herself as a 'fleshy being', after a lifetime of eating disorders and strict regulation of her body. Post-abortion, she experienced kindness and self-love rather than feeling the desire to 'constantly punish' herself (Love, 2021). Similar accounts can be seen in other studies of abortion and embodiment (Broussard, 2020; Siegel, 2020). However, as Link and Phelan (2001, 378) note, 'resistance cannot fully overcome constraint'; accounts of individual resistance to stigma cannot overcome its structural dimensions. Embodiment is clearly a significant element of abortion stigma for some on an individual level. Future work might seek to connect this up more explicitly to the biopolitical dimensions of abortion stigma.

Conclusion

Abortion stigma is a significant feature of individual experiences of abortion, and a broad, discursive, and biopolitical feature of national politics. While a dominant strand of literature conceptualises abortion stigma in individualised, psychological, and quantifiable terms, there is a range of alternative conceptualisations that share an understanding of stigma as an operation of power. Discursive approaches to abortion stigma emphasise its unstable, shifting, and contested nature, through analysis of individual abortion narratives as well as broader political frameworks. An intersectional understanding of abortion stigma resists the call to delineate it from other forms of reproductive stigma, instead placing it in context of marginalisation and oppression through the axes of gender, race, class, and disability. Biopolitical analysis of abortion stigma requires us to think both on the level of individual bodily regulation, and the regulation of the population, and consider how abortion is implicated in nation-building and nationalist imaginaries. Finally, attending to the embodied nature of abortion stigma, thus far neglected in much of the literature, demonstrates the complex interplay of discourse, politics, and the body.

In mapping out the contours of abortion stigma scholarship, I do not conceive of these approaches as mutually exclusive, but instead as mutually reinforcing. Together, they share complementary theoretical traditions and concerns, and build up a conceptualisation of abortion stigma that takes seriously power, oppression, and resistance, and contributes to the wider sociological project of re-politicising stigma as a whole. However, as Kumar (2013) reminds us, not every negative reaction to abortion is stigma. Furthermore, a focus on stigma can assign it too much importance and hinder us from seeing sites of resistance to, or absence of, stigma (Kumar, 2013). Abortion narratives do commonly feature neutral and positive experiences of abortion (Purcell et al, 2020), and 'unapologetic' framings of abortion are also common in some contexts (Baird and Millar, 2019). The ways in which we, as scholars, write about abortion has real effects in the world. Emphasising stigma in the absence of the recognition that abortion brings with it a messy tangle of relief, freedom, joy, sorrow, and care threatens to reify the very problem we seek to contest. The project of conceptualising abortion stigma is, thus, always political.

Could things be different?

- Abortion stigma should be studied not only on the individual and community level, but on institutional, structural, and discursive levels. This would shift the focus for *challenging* stigma from individuals and communities to institutions and States.
- Abortion stigma should be conceptualised in research and activism in relation to power, not only in static, individualised terms as a property one possesses or passes onto others. This would help to understand abortion as part of an explicit 'stigma machine' (Tyler, 2020) that creates consensus around who has a right to reproduce and who has the right to *opt out* of reproduction.
- Research on abortion should move away from concepts of stigma that are limited by narrow psychological reasoning and a reliance on quantitative evidence and, instead, make greater use of discursive, intersectional, biopolitical, and embodied approaches to conceptualising stigma. Research that uses these approaches to understand abortion stigma would be better placed to shed light on stigma's unstable, shifting nature, its relationship to other reproductive stigmas, and how stigma is *felt* by those who experience it.

References

Ahman, E. and Shah, I.H. (2011) 'New estimates and trends regarding unsafe abortion mortality', *International Journal of Gynaecology and Obstetrics*, 115(2): 121–26.

Amy, J.-J. and Rowlands, S. (2018) 'Legalised non-consensual sterilisation – eugenics put into practice before 1945, and the aftermath. Part 1: USA, Japan, Canada and Mexico', *The European Journal of Contraception and Reproductive Health Care*, 23(2): 121–29.

Astbury-Ward, E., Parry, O. and Carnwell, R. (2012) 'Stigma, abortion, and disclosure – Findings from a qualitative study', *Journal of Sexual Medicine*, 9(12): 3137–47.

Baird, B. and Millar, E. (2019) 'More than stigma: Interrogating counter narratives of abortion', *Sexualities*, 22: 1110–26.

Belfrage, M., Ortíz Ramírez, O. and Sorhaindo, A. (2020) 'Story circles and abortion stigma in Mexico: A mixed-methods evaluation of a new intervention for reducing individual level abortion stigma', *Culture, Health and Sexuality*, 22(1): 96–111.

Beynon-Jones, S.M. (2013) 'Expecting motherhood? Stratifying reproduction in 21st-century Scottish abortion practice', *Sociology*, 47(3): 509–25.

Beynon-Jones, S.M. (2017) 'Untroubling abortion: A discourse analysis of women's accounts', *Feminism and Psychology*, 27(2): 225–42.

Biggs, M.A., Upadhyay, U.D., McCulloch, C.E. and Foster, D.G. (2017) 'Women's mental health and well-Being 5 years after receiving or being denied an abortion: A prospective, longitudinal cohort study', *JAMA Psychiatry*, 74(2): 169–78.

Bloomer, F.K., O'Dowd, K. and Macleod, C. (2017) 'Breaking the silence on abortion: The role of adult community abortion education in fostering resistance to norms', *Culture, Health and Sexuality*, 19(7): 709–22.

Boréus, K. (2006) 'Discursive discrimination of the "mentally deficient" in interwar Sweden', *Disability and Society*, 21(5): 441–54.

Broussard, K. (2020) 'The changing landscape of abortion care: Embodied experiences of structural stigma in the Republic of Ireland and Northern Ireland', *Social Science and Medicine*, 245: 112686.

Cárdenas, R., Labandera, A., Baum, S.E., Chiribao, F., Leus, I., Avondet, S. and Friedman, J. (2018) '"It's something that marks you": Abortion stigma after decriminalization in Uruguay', *Reproductive Health*, 15(1): 150.

Center for Reproductive Rights (2022) 'The world's abortion laws', *Center for Reproductive Rights*, [online], Available from: https://reproductiverights.org/maps/worlds-abortion-laws/ [Accessed 7 June 2024].

Cetinkaya, A., Özmen, D., Uyar, F. and Tayhan, A. (2019) 'Reliability and validity of the Turkish version of the Individual-Level Abortion Stigma Scale: A methodological study', *BMJ Open*, 9(4): e024686.

Chen, D., Simons, L., Johnson, E.K., Lockart, B.A. and Finlayson, C. (2017) 'Fertility preservation for transgender adolescents', *Journal of Adolescent Health*, 61(1): 120–3.

Cockrill, K. and Nack, A. (2013) '"I'm not that type of person": Managing the stigma of having an abortion', *Deviant Behaviour*, 34(12): 973–90.

Cockrill, K., Upadhyay, U.D., Turan, J. and Greene Foster, D. (2013) 'The stigma of having an abortion: Development of a scale and characteristics of women experiencing abortion stigma', *Perspectives on Sexual and Reproductive Health*, 45: 79–88.

Colen, S. (1995) '"Like a mother to them": Stratified reproduction and West Indian childcare workers and employers in New York', in F. Ginsburg and R. Rapp (eds), *Conceiving the New World Order: The Global Politics of Reproduction*, Berkeley: University of California Press, pp 78–102.

Crenshaw, K. (1991) 'Mapping the margins: Intersectionality, identity politics, and violence against women of colour', *Stanford Law Review*, 43(6): 1241–99.

Cullen, P. and Korolczuk, E. (2019) 'Challenging abortion stigma: Framing abortion in Ireland and Poland', *Sexual and Reproductive Health Matters*, 27(3): 1686197.

Cutler, A.S., Lundsberg, L.S., White, M.A., Stanwood, N.L. and Gariepy, A.M. (2022) 'The impact of first-person abortion stories on community-level abortion stigma: A randomized trial', *Women's Health Issues*, 32(6): 578–85.

Dunne, P. (2017) 'Transgender sterilisation requirements in Europe', *Medical Law Review*, 25(4): 554–81.

Faundes, A. and Shah, I.H. (2015) 'Evidence supporting broader access to safe legal abortion', *International Journal of Gynaecology and Obstetrics*, 131: S56–9.

Forward Together (2005) 'A new vision for advancing our movement for reproductive health, reproductive rights and reproductive justice', *Forward Together*, [online], Available from: http://forwardtogether.org/assets/docs/ACRJ-A-New-Vision.pdf [Accessed 7 June 2024].

Foucault, M. (1978) *The History of Sexuality Volume I: The Will to Power*, New York: Random House.

Foucault, M. (1998) *The History of Sexuality I: The Will to Knowledge* (new edn), London: Penguin.

Ginsburg, F.D. and Rapp, R. (1995) *Conceiving the New World Order: The Global Politics of Reproduction*, Berkeley: University of California Press.

Goffman, E. (1963) *Stigma: Notes on the Management of Spoiled Identity*, Englewood Cliffs, NJ: Prentice Hall.

Green, L.W. (1988) 'Promoting the one-child policy in China', *Journal of Public Health Policy*, 9(2): 273–83.

Hanschmidt, F., Linde, K., Hilbert, A., Riedel-Heller, S.G. and Kersting, A. (2016) 'Abortion stigma: A systematic review', *Perspectives on Sexual and Reproductive Health*, 48(4): 169–77.

Hanschmidt, F., Nagl, M., Klingner, J., Stepan, H. and Kersting, A. (2018) 'Abortion after diagnosis of fatal anomaly: Psychometric properties of a German version of the individual level abortion stigma scale', *PLOS ONE*, 13(6): e0197986.

Heijnders, M. and Van Der Meij, S. (2006) 'The fight against stigma: An overview of stigma-reduction strategies and interventions', *Psychology, Health and Medicine*, 11(3): 353–63.

Herek, G. (2009) 'Sexual stigma and sexual prejudice in the United States: A conceptual framework', in D. Hope (ed), *Contemporary Perspectives on Lesbian, Gay, and Bisexual Identities*, New York: Springer, pp 65–112.

Hessini, L. (2014) 'A learning agenda for abortion stigma: Recommendations from the Bellagio expert group meeting', *Women and Health*, 54(7): 617–21.

Hill Collins, P. (2002) *Black Feminist Thought: Knowledge, Consciousness, and the Politics of Empowerment* (2nd edn), New York and London: Routledge.

Hoggart, L. (2017) 'Internalised abortion stigma: Young women's strategies of resistance and rejection', *Feminism and Psychology*, 27(2): 186–202.

Hopkins, N., Zeedyk, S. and Raitt, F. (2005) 'Visualising abortion: Emotion discourse and foetal imagery in a contemporary abortion debate', *Social Science and Medicine*, 61(2): 393–403.

Johnson, C. (2008) 'The political "nature" of pregnancy and childbirth', *Canadian Journal of Political Science*, 41(4): 889–913.

Jones, C. (2013) '"Human weeds, not fit to breed?": African Caribbean women and reproductive disparities in Britain', *Critical Public Health*, 23(1): 49–61.

Karaian, L. (2013) 'Pregnant men: Repronormativity, critical trans theory and the re(conceive)ing of sex and pregnancy in law', *Social and Legal Studies*, 22(2): 211–30.

Kimport, K., Foster, K. and Weitz, T.A. (2011) 'Social sources of women's emotional difficulty after abortion: Lessons from women's abortion narratives', *Perspectives on Sexual and Reproductive Health*, 43(2): 103–9.

Kirkman, M., Rowe, H., Hardiman, A. and Rosenthal, D. (2011) 'Abortion is a difficult solution to a problem: A discursive analysis of interviews with women considering or undergoing abortion in Australia', *Women's Studies International Forum*, 34(2): 121–9.

Kumar, A. (2013) 'Everything is not abortion stigma', *Women's Health Issues*, 23(6): e329–31.

Kumar, A., Hessini, L. and Mitchell, E.M.H. (2009) 'Conceptualising abortion stigma', *Culture, Health and Sexuality*, 11(6): 625–39.

Lee, E., Clements, S., Ingham, R. and Stone, N. (2004) *A Matter of Choice? Explaining National Variation in Teenage Abortion and Motherhood*, York: Joseph Rowntree Foundation.

Link, B.G. and Phelan, J.C. (2001) 'Conceptualizing stigma', *Annual Review of Sociology*, 27(1): 363–85.

Love, G. (2021) 'Abortion stigma, class and embodiment in neoliberal England', *Culture, Health and Sexuality*, 23(3): 317–32.

Major, B. and Gramzow, R.H. (1999) 'Abortion as stigma: cognitive and emotional implications of concealment', *Journal of Personality and Social Psychology*, 77(4): 735–45.

Martin, L.A., Hassinger, J.A., Seewald, M. and Harris, L.H. (2018) 'Evaluation of abortion stigma in the workforce: Development of the revised abortion providers stigma scale', *Women's Health Issues*, 28(1): 59–67.

Maternity Care Working Party (2007) 'Making normal birth a reality: Consensus statement from the maternity care working party', *Movimento BH Pelo Parto Normal*, [online], Available from: https://bhpelopartonormal.pbh.gov.br/estudos_cientificos/arquivos/normal_birth_consensus.pdf?__goc_wbp__=205786002x2V4HD1cLqJjwqJYlSxsTTAKB3w [Accessed 7 June 2024].

McNay, L. (1991) 'The Foucauldian body and the exclusion of experience', *Hypatia*, 6(3): 125–39.

Millar, E. (2020) 'Abortion stigma as a social process', *Women's Studies International Forum*, 78: 102328.

Mishtal, J. (2012) 'Irrational non-reproduction? The "dying nation" and the postsocialist logics of declining motherhood in Poland', *Anthropology and Medicine*, 19(2): 153–69.

MYA Network (n.d.) 'The issue of tissue', *MYA Network*, [online], Available from: https://myanetwork.org/the-issue-of-tissue/ [Accessed 7 June 2024].

Nixon, L. (2013) 'The right to (trans) parent: A reproductive justice approach to reproductive rights, fertility, and family-building issues facing transgender people', *William and Mary Journal of Women and the Law*, 20(1): 73–103.

Ó Cionnaith, F. (2018) 'Referendum vote is "Ireland's second chance": Leo Varadkar's speech in full', *Irish Examiner*, [online] 26 May, Available from: https://www.irishexaminer.com/opinion/commentanalysis/arid-30845292.html [Accessed 7 June 2024].

Parker, R. and Aggleton, P. (2003) 'HIV and AIDS-related stigma and discrimination: A conceptual framework and implications for action', *Social Science and Medicine*, 57(1): 13–24.

Pegoraro, L. (2015) 'Second-rate victims: The forced sterilization of Indigenous peoples in the USA and Canada', *Settler Colonial Studies*, 5(2): 161–73.

Petchesky, R.P. (1990) *Abortion and Woman's Choice: The State, Sexuality, and Reproductive Freedom*, Boston, MA: Northeastern University Press.

Purcell, C., Brown, A., Melville, C. and McDaid, L.M. (2017) 'Women's embodied experiences of second trimester medical abortion', *Feminism and Psychology*, 27(2): 163–85.

Purcell, C., Hilton, S. and McDaid, L. (2014) 'The stigmatisation of abortion: A qualitative analysis of print media in Great Britain in 2010', *Culture, Health and Sexuality*, 16(9): 1141–55.

Purcell, C., Maxwell, K., Bloomer, F., Rowlands, S. and Hoggart, L. (2020) 'Toward normalising abortion: Findings from a qualitative secondary analysis study', *Culture, Health and Sexuality*, 22(12): 1349–64.

Repo, J. (2019) 'Governing juridical sex: Gender recognition and the biopolitics of trans sterilization in Finland', *Politics and Gender*, 15(1): 83–106.

Roberti, A. (2021) '"Women deserve better:" The use of the pro-woman frame in anti-abortion policies in U.S. states', *Journal of Women, Politics and Policy*, 42(3): 207–24.

Rocca, C.H., Moseson, H., Gould, H., Foster, D.G. and Kimport, K. (2021) 'Emotions over five years after denial of abortion in the United States: Contextualizing the effects of abortion denial on women's health and lives', *Social Science and Medicine*, 269: 113567.

Sanger, C. (2017) *About Abortion: Terminating Pregnancy in Twenty-First Century America*, Cambridge, MA and London: The Belknap Press of Harvard University Press.

Save the 8th (n.d.) 'Campaign launch: Vote no', *Heroes*, [online], Available from: https://www.save8.ie/the_campaign/campaign-launch-vote-no/ [Accessed 7 June 2024].

Scambler, G. (2018) 'Heaping blame on shame: "Weaponising stigma" for neoliberal times', *The Sociological Review*, 66(4): 766–82.

Shakespeare, T. (1998) 'Choices and rights: Eugenics, genetics and disability equality', *Disability and Society*, 13(5): 665–81.

Sheldon, S. (1997) *Beyond Control: Medical Power, Women and Abortion Law*, London: Pluto Press.

Shellenberg, K.M., Moore, A.M., Bankole, A., Juarez, F., Omideyi, A.K., Palomino, N. et al (2011) 'Social stigma and disclosure about induced abortion: Results from an exploratory study', *Global Public Health*, 6(Suppl 1): S111–25.

Shilling, C. (2007) *The Body and Social Theory*, Oxford: Blackwell.

Siegel, D.P. (2020) 'Medicalization and naturalization: Understanding abortion as a naturecultural phenomenon', *Catalyst: Feminism, Theory, Technoscience*, 6(2).

Silliman, J.M. (2004) *Undivided Rights: Women of Color Organize for Reproductive Justice*, Cambridge, MA: South End Press.

Simpson, A.V., Clegg, S.R., Lopes, M.P., e Cunha, M.P., Rego, A. and Pitsis, T. (2014) 'Doing compassion or doing discipline? Power relations and the Magdalene Laundries', *Journal of Political Power*, 7(2): 253–74.

SisterSong Collective (n.d.) 'Reproductive justice', *SisterSong, Inc*, [online], Available from: http://sistersong.net/reproductive-justice/ [Accessed 7 June 2024].

Skeggs, B. (1997) *Formations of Class and Gender: Becoming Respectable*, London and Thousand Oaks, CA: SAGE Publications Ltd.

Skeggs, B. (2004) *Class, Self, Culture*, London: Routledge.

Sorhaindo, A.M., Karver, T.S., Karver, J.G. and Garcia, S.G. (2016) 'Constructing a validated scale to measure community-level abortion stigma in Mexico', *Contraception*, 93(5): 421–31.

Together For Yes (n.d.) 'Real stories archive', [online]', Available from: https://www.togetherforyes.ie/real-stories/ [Accessed 7 June 2024].

Tyler, I. (2008) '"Chav mum chav scum": Class disgust in contemporary Britain', *Feminist Media Studies*, 8(1): 17–34.

Tyler, I. (2020) *Stigma: The Machinery of Inequality*, London: Zed Books.

Tyler, I. and Slater, T. (2018) 'Rethinking the sociology of stigma', *The Sociological Review*, 66(4): 721–43.

Vergès, F. (2018) 'On women and their wombs: Capitalism, racialization, feminism', *Critical Times*, 1(1): 263–7.

Weissman, A.L. (2017) 'Repronormativity and the reproduction of the nation-state: The state and sexuality collide', *Journal of GLBT Family Studies*, 13(3): 277–305.

Williams, O. and Annandale, E. (2020) 'Obesity, stigma and reflexive embodiment: Feeling the "weight" of expectation', *Health*, 24(4), 421–41.

Wyatt, D. and Hughes, K. (2009) 'When discourse defies belief: Anti-abortionists in contemporary Australia', *Journal of Sociology*, 45(3): 235–53.

Yuval-Davis, N. (1996) 'Women and the biological reproduction of "the nation"', *Women's Studies International Forum*, 19(1–2): 17–24.

4

Shooting Blanks? Exploring the Assumed Relationship Between Masculinity and Stigma in Male Fertility

Esmée Hanna, Caroline Law, and Nicky Hudson

Introduction

Male infertility is often considered to be a source of stigma for men (Hanna and Gough, 2015), with assumptions that men experience greater stigma in relation to fertility issues than women (Gannon et al, 2004). The stigmatisation from infertility is linked with hegemonic masculinity – considered the most 'ideal' way to be a man (Connell, 1995) – specifically around the value placed on men being both virile and fertile (Inhorn, 2004). Yet, in research to date, evidence for stigma being explicitly examined in relation to male infertility is limited (Gannon et al, 2004; Hanna and Gough, 2015). After offering a consideration of how stigma may be defined, this chapter explores how fertility and masculinity are intertwined and how, in this context, male infertility has been perceived to cause stigma. We argue that ideas of masculinity, virility, and fertility have become problematically co-constituted, whereby if a man is infertile, his sexual capacity and potency, and his masculinity, are called into question. We also argue that there is insufficient research evidence which demonstrates and unpacks how exactly stigma operates in cases of male infertility. The chapter concludes with a call for future research to explore the intersections of masculinities, infertility, and stigma, which considers the experiences and perspectives of men – in order to more meaningfully understand how stigma operates in relation to male infertility. Such research would then provide a robust and meaningful basis for us to begin to tackle and challenge any such stigma.

Defining stigma

Stigma is an often-used concept within sociology, but a precise definition can be elusive, especially as it is utilised across different contexts and areas of study (Link and Phelan, 2001). As Link and Phelan (2001) note, there is also a vast array of research on stigma (LeBel, 2008), but of this work, there is much that fails to ever explicitly define or introduce a working definition of stigma. Sociologist Erving Goffman (1963, 3) is famously credited with influencing sociological understandings of stigma, defining it as 'an attribute that is deeply discrediting'. This seemingly pithy definition has since been expanded and extended. Link and Phelan (2001), for example, offer a much longer explanation of stigma that emphasises how stigma involves multiple aspects which are connected and active in relation to one another. This positions stigmatisation as a social process. Similarly, LeBel (2008, 410–11) suggests that 'it is generally understood that members of stigmatized groups are devalued and discriminated against by the general public and often suffer from social exclusion and status loss as a result'. Both Link and Phelan's (2001) and LeBel's (2008) conceptualisations of stigma, which foreground the labelling and devaluing of human differences and subsequent status loss and social exclusion, show how social processes interact to create stigma. It is this conceptualisation that informs our thinking in this chapter. If we accept that stigma is rooted in the social identification of human differences, this leads us to question whether and how stigma occurs when men's fertility experiences differ from accepted norms of fertility and procreation – and to question how contextual factors relating to fertility and masculinity may shape this.

The portrayal of stigma in relation to male infertility

'Urban Dictionary' – a crowdsourced site which defines contemporary slang – includes the following entry: 'Jaffa: A male who can't produce sperm, Jaffa being derived from the title of a fruit company whose Oranges are seedless'. Colloquial 'jokes' of men 'being Jaffas', thereby being 'seedless', illuminate the way in which fertility and masculinity are seen as being intrinsically and problematically intertwined; 'throughout history and across cultures, the ideal macho man is depicted as virile and potent' (Barnes, 2014, 4). This is particularly the case in a heteronormative culture, that is, a culture that assumes being heterosexual is 'normal', correct, and default, and which is organised and operates with cisgendered, heterosexual people's needs and lives prioritised. The importance of 'sowing seed' as the means of creating new life is evident in biblical references as well as in cultural representations in contemporary society, indicating its pervasiveness over time. Some argue that the 'seed metaphor' reconfigured notions of reproductive power, seeing those with the seed (men) as the holder of power; and that this conceptualisation set the course of gendered dynamics and the subordination of women through to the present day (McElvaine, 2017). Indeed, the Latin for 'seed' is 'semen', with something 'seminal' correspondingly defined as being important. What it means to be a man, to be powerful, is therefore routinely aligned with what it means to be fertile.

Many societies remain keenly pro-natalist, meaning they place high value on fertility and parenthood (Gannon et al, 2004). This creates a context in which wanting to have children is expected, though not equally. While parenthood is socially mandated for groups with high levels of social and cultural capital, the situation is reversed for socially excluded and marginalised communities (Culley et al, 2009). Against this backdrop, the inability to have children is seen to cause shame for those affected. This is particularly so when the cause is male factor infertility (that is, where the fertility 'problem' is found in the male-sexed body, usually relating to having no/low sperm or poor-quality sperm). In her book *Conceiving Masculinity*, Barnes (2014) details the numerous myths which surround male infertility, highlighting how misunderstandings shape the experience. Recent years have seen greater research into the experience of male infertility including, importantly, from the perspective of men themselves (Hanna and Gough, 2015, 2016, 2017, 2020), but there is some way to go to truly operationalise and understand the relationship between stigma and infertility.

Contemporary research in reproduction gives us greater insight into the feelings men themselves may have about fertility issues. Recent work discusses how the need to use donor sperm, due to male factor infertility, creates a heightened sense of stigma and shame for infertile men, in part due to men's perceptions of sperm donors being more 'potent' (Cosson et al, 2022). In keeping with LeBel's (2008) definition of stigma, which foregrounds the devaluing of difference and the status loss that occurs as a result, the casting of fertility/infertility as a success/failure binary is seen as contributing to the possibility of stigma. Being seen to have 'failed' in something which society prizes has the potential to contribute to men feeling shame in the context of their infertility. Research with men experiencing infertility highlights the complex emotions that men describe, including a sense of stigma (Hanna and Gough, 2020).

Men also report that fertility clinics feel highly female-focused and that some fertility practitioners lack empathy, thereby contributing to men feeling they are a separate group and having a sense of being 'other' (Hanna and Gough, 2020). Descriptions of the crushing grief, the falling into obsessions (be it with work or extramarital sex to bolster their sense of self), and the isolation of infertility all demonstrate the significance that experiencing infertility has for men. Rome's (2020) work on men's blogs about infertility shows how men experience grief and shame as infertility destabilises their sense of masculinity. Sharing their 'wounded bodies' online means they must navigate the stigma of their experience and present themselves as vulnerable, albeit this may be temporary in the hope of ultimately recovering their sense of masculinity (Rome, 2020).

Silence is often seen as a central feature of stigma and shame. In a study by Cosson et al (2022) with heterosexual men who had used donor sperm, participants rarely wanted to tell others about their use of a donor, including their donor-conceived children. Allison (2011, 1) highlights how the negative impacts of silence are powerful and pervasive:

> Silence is both imposed and embraced. While it is sometimes self-imposed and purposeful, the pervasive presence of silence amplifies the suffering of many individuals and couples who are infertile. Silence serves to obscure from view much of the experience of infertility, ostensibly to protect privacy while at the same time occluding opportunities to promote a wider public understanding of what it means to be infertile.

Daniels (2006, 70) suggests that this silence has been systematised via a lack of medical research into male reproductive issues, which is in part due to the social denial of male infertility and reluctance to see male fertility as requiring medical 'treatment':

> As long as male reproductive function was symbolic of manhood and male vulnerability was a source of shame, few men would stand up to demand public attention to the issues. Scientists, physicians and politicians fed this reservoir of shame by their reluctance to adequately examine questions of male reproductive health.

In seeking to explore the co-constitution of stigma and male infertility, we need to consider when and how male infertility becomes visible or not, and how significant these ideas and expectations are for culturally dominant ideas about what it means to be a man. It is towards these considerations which this chapter turns next.

Hegemonic masculinity

> We need only suggest the converse of current ideals of manhood to see the power such ideals still hold in our cultural imagination: men are weak, men are vulnerable, men are impotent, needy and dependent. This is the image not of a man but of an 'effeminate'. It is an image of the end of manhood, the antithesis of masculinity. (Daniels, 2006, 158)

Masculinity is the socially valorised ideal of what it means to be a man. The quote from Daniels neatly recognises deeply rooted ideas about how men should and should not behave, and what makes a *real man*. To understand the way in which masculinities continue to be central to the way we understand the perceived stigma around infertility, we need to look more closely at how power differences exist between men and women, and between different groups of men. One of the most significant contributions to the understanding of masculinities comes from the writings of Connell (1995). Connell's work has developed sociological insights into how power operates to enable a patriarchal society, where men are positioned as dominant, powerful, and in control of how men's needs and requirements become prioritised:

> Hegemonic masculinity was understood as the pattern of practice (i.e., things done, not just a set of role expectations or an identity) that allowed men's dominance over women to continue. Hegemonic masculinity was distinguished from other masculinities, especially subordinated masculinities. Hegemonic masculinity was not assumed to be normal in the statistical sense; only a minority of men might enact it. But it was certainly normative. It embodied the currently most honoured way of being a man, it required all other men to position themselves in relation to it, and it ideologically legitimated the global subordination of women to men. (Connell and Messerschmidt, 2005, 832)

Hegemonic masculinity is, therefore, not something that is lived or enacted by all men, but rather something which society proffers as a benchmark against which men (and women) are then positioned and judged. The characteristics of masculinity that are valued by this notion of hegemonic masculinity include: physical strength and a muscular physique; dominance; sexual prowess (both virile and fertile); and self-control and mastery of emotions (Burton, 2014). We can also see in the opposite of these ideals the construction of femininity as encapsulating weakness, dependency, submission, and emotional expression. The socialisation of boys inducts them into these normative ideals, and inevitably many men find they are unable to live up to a largely unattainable model. It is in the mismatch between the norms of hegemonic masculinity on the one hand, and men's individual opportunities to meet these ideals on the other, that we can begin to see vulnerabilities in self-identity arise. As Barnes (2014, 7) notes, '[i]n reality, the achievement of perfect manhood and masculinity is possible for only a small, privileged minority. As a result, most men suffer from feelings of powerlessness and inadequacy'.

Within the conceptualisation of hegemonic masculinity, others have articulated how Connell (1995) suggests that multiple masculinities exist and that other non-hegemonic masculinities are themselves important in considering the way in which hegemonic masculinity is constructed and upheld (Messerschmidt, 2019a). It is important to note that hegemonic masculinity is viewed as relational; central to its hierarchical nature is its connection within and between groups (Gough, 2018). One of the major enduring criticisms of theories of hegemonic masculinity, however, is the notion that it can reinforce the idea that masculine traits are natural and inevitable for men (Gough, 2018). In contemporary theorising, several new ideas and theories about how masculinity works have been offered, which are explored later in this chapter. However, hegemonic masculinity remains a constant feature, even if only to arrange alternative gender identities. For that reason, it remains useful to first examine the perceived interrelation of hegemonic masculinity and infertility.

Fertility and virility: the meeting point of hegemonic masculinity?

Contemporary society positions hegemonic masculinity as the ideal way of being a man, and as part of this construction, the notion of virility – comprising sexual strength, drive, and energy – is upheld as one of the most important traits of manhood. Further, virility and fertility are often conflated; they are considered one and the same (the so-called 'fertility–virility linkage' [Lloyd, 1996]). Within a heteronormative culture, a man capable of sexual 'conquest' of women is, therefore, assumed to be capable of fathering children. Conversely, not only does an individual man's inability to have children call into question his sexual prowess, but the possibility of men being vulnerable in the reproductive arena may also call into question manhood itself. As such, the common conflation of virility and fertility exacerbates the potential for infertility stigma.

Given the dominance of hegemonic masculinity within gender relations, it remains socially beneficial within a patriarchal society to ensure that fertility and reproduction are seen as the domain of women and to perpetuate the myth that men are immune from weakness, including reproductive 'failings' (Daniels, 2006). The stigma suggested to be associated with male infertility can, therefore, be seen as due to the perceived 'deviance' of infertile men from the ideal of hegemonic masculinity, highlighting an 'example of masculinity going wrong' (de Boer, 2022, 148). Societies in which hegemonic masculinity is highly prized may also be strongly pro-natalist, exacerbating male infertility as problematic:

> People should reproduce; moreover, they should want to reproduce. When one is infertile, what are the purposes of heterosexual marriage, sexual intercourse, and even life? In a culture in which virility is

synonymous with masculinity and fertility is often conflated with virility, what does it mean to be an infertile man? (Barnes, 2014, 84–5)

In this sense, failure to conceive is a sexual failure; the purpose of the act itself is defeated. Importantly, this applies specifically to heterosexual men. Queer people may automatically 'fail' this test of sexual relations being a necessary component of successful conception. The experiences of queer people regarding infertility, and specifically if and how stigma features in these experiences, is also under-researched (but it is not the primary focus here).

Daniels (2006, 164) moves beyond positioning the perceived 'weakness' of infertility as problematic for individuals by suggesting instead that presenting men as 'invulnerable' to reproductive harm has wider biopolitical motivations and implications: 'The health of the male body remains symbolic of the health of the nation, with sperm counts a measure of national virility. The nation is weakened by the image of weakened men.' Whether such biopolitical consequences can be inferred is perhaps a subject for elsewhere, but it does serve to illuminate the levels of importance that may be attached to both fertility and hegemonic masculinity – and how a failure to achieve conception is constructed as a more wide-ranging failure of masculinity, kinship, or of nation itself.

The idea that infertility arises from issues of sexual performance is not new. Such ideas were identified in the 1980s as being a central reason that male infertility was not being researched, due to it being seen as 'taboo' (Bents, 1985). This longstanding myth is often based on assumptions that infertile men have less testosterone so are 'less biologically manly' (Barnes, 2014, 87). While the boon of Viagra may have reduced some of the stigma around erectile dysfunction (Vares et al, 2003), the notion of poor sexual function is still routinely viewed as problematic by and for men in relation to masculinity. It has been suggested that the centrality of sexual performance in hegemonic masculinity is due to the 'ejaculation imperative': 'The ability to ejaculate, the quantity of semen produced, and the forcefulness of their ejaculation all become the hallmark of a hegemonic masculine ideal, to which males aspire' (Johnson, 2010, 239).

The importance of ejaculation for both conception and masculinity shows the conflation of fertility and virility, and the centrality of heterosexuality within that. De Boer's (2022) exploration of fictionalised accounts of male infertility highlights the fertility–virility linkage as one of the four core themes of how infertility is presented in contemporary media. However, de Boer (2022) concludes that men's hegemonic masculinity is always restored in the plotlines of television dramas, perhaps reinforcing the notion that infertility is, at best, a temporary challenge to masculinity that can be overcome, rather than something which can characterise the lives of men across their life-course.

Conflating fertility and sexual performance contribute to the perception of infertile men as being 'deficient' in a key component of hegemonic masculinity (Gannon et al, 2004). A recent article in *Men's Health* magazine described male fertility issues as the 'last great sexual taboo' (Manzoor, 2019), demonstrating how ingrained such notions are and why male infertility may remain stigmatised. It raises the question of whether what is perceived to be problematic is men's inability to have children or the sexual impotency that is assumed or inferred from male infertility. However, limited research has attempted to unravel this conflation of infertility and impotence, which hampers our understandings of stigma in this context. The following section takes a closer examination of how the research on male infertility has engaged with ideas of stigma, but arguably has failed to do so in a meaningful way.

The explicit evidence of stigma

As discussed, fertility (in part due to its conflation with virility) is seen as a central feature of hegemonic masculinity, with infertility resulting in a discrediting of masculinity. Goffman's (1963) classic work on stigma suggests that stigma spoils the identities of those who become stigmatised, discrediting them and setting them apart from the rest of society (Cook and Dickens, 2014). It is important to also note that Goffman himself did not directly discuss infertility in relation to stigma, although as Whiteford and Gonzalez (1995, 29) note in their work on women's experiences of infertility and stigma, Goffman cited work which 'equated infertility to being crippled'.

Stigma is rarely the central focus of research on male infertility and is, instead, often a secondary consideration as part of work on masculinity (Inhorn, 2003; Barnes, 2014; Dolan at al, 2017; Hanna and Gough, 2022). Work focusing on stigma and infertility includes that of Gannon et al (2004), whose central conclusion was that male infertility is stigmatised due to the conflation with virility. Their work is one example whereby stigma is a central focus, but where the mechanics of how such stigma operates are left unspecified. In focusing on media portrayals of declining male fertility rates, Gannon et al (2004) explore the cultural discourses around male infertility, but do not specifically illuminate the experiences of men themselves. Inhorn's (2004) study of experiences of male infertility in the Middle East – unique in focusing on experiences outside of the Euro-American context – demonstrates the complex interrelation of technology, culture, religion, and gender identity with stigma. In the Middle East, male infertility is considered to be highly emasculating, and Inhorn (2004) describes how reproductive technologies – such as IVF (in vitro fertilisation) – may change the social visibility of male infertility by making pregnancy possible, and thereby masking male infertility from public view. Inhorn's work aside, much of the research on male infertility, including that exploring the experience and negotiation of stigma, focuses often on cis, heterosexual, white men. Interrogations of race, class, and age are largely absent from such enquiries (Cervi and Knights, 2022).

The existing literature on male infertility, therefore, proposes that stigma results due to the challenges infertility poses to masculinity and the 'deficiencies' it illuminates. This raises an important question of whether 'emasculation' is the same as 'stigmatisation'. In the absence of research which considers how emasculation and stigma operate in relation to infertility, work from complementary areas helps to further our understanding. Work on erectile dysfunction has examined the connection between emasculation and stigma through the lens of 'honour based' cultures (Foster et al, 2022). In such contexts, men's reputations are seen as being built through endorsing norms which align to characteristics central to hegemonic masculinity, including sexual virility. In their work, Foster et al describe how a man's inability to display sexual conquest of women, because of erectile dysfunction, is experienced as a source of 'dishonour' and, therefore, potentially damaging to their sense of self. 'Honour-endorsing' men, they claim, show higher levels of stigma regarding erectile dysfunction, whereby men who 'buy into' the norms of masculinity are more likely to experience phenomena which are 'threats' to masculinity as a form of stigma. Foster et al also discuss how, in cases of erectile dysfunction, there is the potential for honour to be re-established, in that virility can, through medical treatment, be restored.

In contrast, one of Goffman's central contributions on stigma was that '[h]e showed how a spoiled identity could rarely be redeemed because it denies stigmatized individuals an opportunity to present themselves to others and to society as they might justly be entitled to appear' (Cook and Dickens, 2014, 89). This is a further complexity in the case of male infertility and stigma, since it raises questions about whether the spoiled identity can be redeemed if conception does occur, either through treatment such as IVF or *naturally*. If we see IVF as *fixing* infertility, this suggests that infertility-related stigma may also not be fixed, but potentially reversible or mutable. However, for men with azoospermia (men who have no sperm), this is never going to be possible.

In the limited literature on male infertility that discusses stigma, few engage with wider theory around stigma itself. Marcia Inhorn's (2004) work is one example where Goffman's work on stigma is used. Inhorn uses the concept to set up the context of male infertility in the Middle East, but this is not pulled through into theoretical conclusions regarding stigma itself. Work that provides a more detailed and theoretically informed interrogation of infertility-associated stigma tends to focus on women and female factor infertility (Remennick, 2000; Riessman, 2000; Whiteford and Gonzalez, 1995). This work shows that stigma for women is due to the inability to follow the life-pattern expected of them, and that deviating from this expectation to reproduce is more problematic within pro-natalist societies. As Whiteford and Gonzalez (1995, 29) write, women 'feel as though they have broken some accepted, if unspoken, cultural rule and they pay for it by being classified as "other". Infertile women refer to their fertile sisters as "normals"'.

While focusing on the female experience, the work that does exist on the stigma of infertility offers further insight into the possible connections between infertility and stigma for men. That there is limited literature attending directly to an analysis of men's experiences of infertility in relation to stigma highlights how a concept such as stigma is often used, but frequently under-evidenced. Indeed, it relies on the assumptions that 'deficiencies' in masculinity automatically result in stigma. Yet, scholars of men and masculinities suggest that ideas of what constitute 'deficiencies' in masculinities, and indeed what it means to be a man more generally, may be shifting.

Changing masculinities

The assumption that failure to live up to hegemonic norms of masculinity equates to stigma rests on the idea that hegemonic masculinity is still held up as the ideal way to be a man in contemporary society. Barnes (2014, 8) notes that '[m]ale infertility provides a useful case study for exploring masculine themes because infertility prevents men from accomplishing the most hegemonic form of masculinity'. It is therefore important, in attempting to unravel the interconnections between stigma and infertility, that we also take time to assess how and in what ways masculinities may (or may not) be changing. One of the core criticisms of Connell's (1995) conceptualisation of hegemonic masculinity is that it can reinforce ideas that masculine traits are natural and inevitable for men and, in doing so, makes masculinity appear as fixed and unaffected by wider cultural changes. In recent years, a range of ideas and theories in relation to understanding masculinities have been presented, including inclusive masculinities (Anderson, 2010), caring masculinities (Elliot, 2016), hybrid masculinities (Bridges and Pascoe, 2014), emergent masculinities (Inhorn, 2012), and liquid masculinities (Hanna and Gough, 2022). This multiplicity of theory can be viewed as the 'third phase' of research on men and masculinities, characterised by plurality being a key characteristic (Hearn et al, 2012). While substantial differences between these various theories exist, central to many of them is the notion that, within contemporary societies, we see men doing masculinities in many different ways. We can therefore see 'contemporary masculinities as evolving, convoluted and rich, with men grappling with conventional and modern ideals and practices relating to their bodies, emotions and relationship with self and others' (Gough, 2018, 75).

While many authors, Gough included, see cautious optimism about progressive changes in ideas about what it means to 'be a man', many of these new masculinities theories do not see hegemonic masculinity as redundant (Lohan, 2015). Male social dominance, gender inequity, and heteronormativity remain stubbornly evident in many contemporary and apparently 'progressive' societies. Nonetheless, many of those working in the space of men and masculinities do point to the 'progress and possibilities' that we are now seeing (Gough, 2018).

We know, for example, that some men are happy to share their feelings related to infertility (albeit within particular contexts) (Hanna and Gough, 2016), that many men make substantial changes to their lives due to their commitment to seeking to become fathers (Hanna et al, 2018; Hanna and Gough, 2022), and that they reach out and both seek and offer support and help to and from other men about fertility issues (Hanna and Gough, 2018). This is not to say that, within certain contexts, 'traditional' scripts that draw on hegemonic masculine expectations, such as stoicism, strength, and mastery of emotions, are not still highly evident (Throsby and Gill, 2004). But alongside this growing visibility and awareness of men's experiences of infertility through documentaries, films, comedy, and public figures sharing their own experiences is beginning to cast light into an aspect of men's lives previously kept hidden from the public gaze. We see the media increasingly open to a 'new' modelling of masculinity, where men's openness with their 'personal struggles' is seen as something to be lauded rather than a source of shame (Hansen, 2022).

What, then, does this mean for stigma in relation to infertility? If we take that the presentation of masculinities may well be changing, so that the dominance of hegemonic forms of masculinity is weaker, it should follow that stigma arising from a range of issues seen to be at odds with hegemonic masculinity (such as infertility) should also be declining. Yet, research, including our own, still points to men discussing shame and stigma related to infertility (Hanna and Gough, 2020), as well as medical professionals' attempts to spare men the 'shame' seen as associated with infertility (Barnes, 2014). How fixed the experience of stigma may be in this context is, therefore, dependent on several aspects, including how meaningful and widespread changes in masculinities are.

Messerschmidt's (2019b) definition of 'positive masculinities' is particularly helpful here. Messerschmidt offers a clear depiction of alternative masculinities as being 'counter hegemonic' (that is, actively challenging the value placed on hegemonic masculinity) and as contributing to seeking greater equality between men and women, and between different groups of men. This is, however, notably different from performative or 'micro' aspects of 'softer masculinities', which are still, in fact, embedded within long-standing ideas about the importance of hegemonic masculinity, and the power imbalances and inequality it perpetuates: '[P]ractices that previously were identified as feminine behaviour became recognized and established as positive masculine behaviour and thus challenged gender hegemony' (Messerschmidt, 2019b, 28). For infertility, this remains challenging, as an experience known to be distressing is unlikely to be incorporated as positive behaviour. However, open expressions of emotion (traditionally positioned as a feminine trait), including expressions of disappointment and distress arising from infertility, could potentially be established as a positive behaviour.

Looking beyond infertility, we have seen considerable shifts in what it means to be a father in recent years, with men more openly expressing their desire to be fathers (Hadley, 2020), emotionally investing in family life (Morman and Floyd, 2002), and embracing involved, intimate fatherhood (Dermott, 2008, Dermott and Miller, 2015, Lohan, 2015). Such trends, while potentially evidence of positive masculine behaviours, may have the potential to heighten the stigma of infertility. For example, they reinforce pro-natalist ideas about how having children, and wanting to have children, is natural and normal. In this context, not being able to have children may still be highly problematic. On the other hand, we also know there are changes in how people think about and choose to do family life (Christofidou, 2021), with increasing numbers of people opting to remain childless by choice (Smith et al, 2020). Whether these aspects are sufficiently significant to alter the experience of infertility stigma – to reduce it by decentring the importance of parenthood in the life-course – remains highly uncertain. As scholars of men and masculinities have noted, those with privilege often have much greater choice in gender expression. Indeed, some changes in the expression of masculinities does not mean that *all* men are experiencing such changes (Christofidou, 2021).

Conclusion

In working through what we know about the connections between masculinities and stigma in relation to infertility, the notion of 'shooting blanks' seems apt. We are attempting to unravel an experience, but with insufficient insights on which to base this. That so little research has directly and explicitly focused on men, fertility, and stigma is telling. This is not to say that existing discussion within infertility research of how men experience stigma is to be dismissed, but often it is the by-product of research into the infertility experience as a whole, rather than the specific focus. Where stigma is discussed, it is rarely defined, conceptualised, or considered in a theoretically meaningful way. Even though many scholars suggest that there are changes to the nature of masculinities, the impact of these potentially positive 'micro' shifts are perhaps not being followed through in explorations of their meaning or impact at the macro level. As Christofidou (2021, 10) notes, '[t]he tolerance or incorporation of stigmatised elements does not mean abandonment of hegemonic power'. Beginning to unpack the deeper connections between gender norms and stigma would, thus, be pertinent to understand if any such abandonment of hegemonic power is visible within new forms of masculinities. But to do so, more substantive empirical knowledge is needed.

A more concerted effort to understand what, if any, impact stigma from infertility has in the lives of men directly, as well as to attempt to gain men's own perspectives on how the fertility–virility linkage features in their experience of infertility and stigma, would undoubtedly advance our understandings, particularly if focused on relational and intersectional aspects. Much of the research on men and masculinities, and specifically its theorising, is focused on high-income Global North countries, but then applied universally to the rest of the world. The nuance and differences of class, culture, ethnicity, and sexuality all need to be more openly considered in relation to men's experiences of infertility and stigma. We know, for example, that in the Global North, minoritised ethnic groups may experience greater stigma around reproduction than white men (Culley et al, 2013). Yet, too often, we do not hear the voices of these men in reproduction research. In exploring stigma and infertility for men, we therefore need to move beyond assumptions on several levels to more carefully understand how, or indeed if, stigma is encountered by men experiencing infertility. We also have an opportunity to better understand what the experience (or not) of stigma may tell us about the nature of masculinities and social expectations of men more broadly.

What, then, does the analysis of male infertility and stigma offered in this chapter mean for our understandings of stigma more generally? As this chapter suggests, a theoretically informed, nuanced, in-depth consideration of if and how stigma operates in the context of male infertility is lacking. This begs the question, in what other fields of sociology, and in relation to what other social phenomena, is stigma unquestioningly assumed? Have, in some contexts, 'common sense' assumptions of the inevitability of stigma eclipsed a more critical questioning – and does this call for a 'rescuing' of stigma theory? The ways in which stigma is a kind of 'absent presence' in scholarship on male infertility suggests that, in some contexts, there may be a need for stigma theory to be revisited, reapplied, and recalibrated.

Could things be different?

Many of the issues discussed in this chapter require a change in focus, as well as attitudes and assumptions, so that things may change. If, on further exploration and assessment, stigma is still seen to be inherent within the experience of male infertility, then we suggest that change may be made by:

- Having a greater visibility of male infertility and breaking down the silence and secrecy surrounding infertility. The media is well-placed to do this by showcasing the experiences of men who are infertile in stories, dramas, films, and comedy, so that it becomes a 'normal', accepted part of social life.
- Ensuring greater reproductive education so that there is wider understanding that fertility and virility, and therefore infertility and impotence, are not the same. Tackling stigma around impotence for men would also help reduce the correlated stigma that infertility receives.
- Researching men's experiences of infertility using an intersectional approach – that is, exploring how experiences of infertility and stigma may vary across socioeconomic groups, by sexuality and gender identity, and (dis)ability. This should include research outside of dominant groups in the Global North to learn more about men's experiences of infertility in the Global South and those of men from minoritised ethnic groups. Such research would provide a robust and meaningful basis for us to begin to tackle and challenge any stigma found to be associated with male infertility in a meaningful and culturally informed way.
- Shifting cultural norms associated with gender, especially as they relate to men and masculinities, to include greater acceptance of a range of different ways of being a man. This will require greater social support for and promotion of non-traditional expressions of gender and tackling the power imbalances between women and men to create more equal societies.

References

Allison, J. (2011) 'Conceiving silence: Infertility as discursive contradiction in Ireland', *Medical Anthropology Quarterly,* 25(1): 1–21.

Anderson, E. (2010), *Inclusive Masculinity: The Changing Nature of Masculinities,* London: Routledge.

Barnes, L.W. (2014) *Conceiving Masculinity: Male Infertility, Medicine, and Identity,* Philadelphia: Temple University Press.

Bents, H. (1985) 'Psychology of male infertility – A literature survey', *International Journal of Andrology,* 8(4): 325–36.

Bridges, T. and Pascoe, C.J. (2014) 'Hybrid masculinities: New directions in the sociology of men and masculinities', *Sociology Compass,* 8(3): 246–58.

Burton, M. (2014) 'Negotiating masculinity: How infertility impacts hegemonic masculinity', *Laurier Undergraduate Journal of the Arts*, 1(1): 49–57.

Cervi, L. and Knights, D. (2022) 'Organizing male infertility: Masculinities and fertility treatment', *Gender, Work and Organization*, 29(4): 1113–31.

Christofidou, A. (2021) 'Men and masculinities: A continuing debate on change', *NORMA*, 16(2): 81–97.

Cook, R.J. and Dickens, B.M. (2014) 'Reducing stigma in reproductive health', *International Journal of Gynaecology and Obstetrics*, 125(1): 89–92.

Connell, R.W. (1995) *Masculinities*, Cambridge: Polity Press.

Connell, R.W. and Messerschmidt, J.W. (2005) 'Hegemonic masculinity: Rethinking the concept', *Gender and Society*, 19(6): 829–59.

Cosson, B., Dempsey, D. and Kelly, F. (2022) 'Secret shame – Male infertility and donor conception in the wake of retrospective legislative change', *Men and Masculinities*, 25(3): 497–515.

Culley, L., Hudson, N. and Lohan, M. (2013) 'Where are all the men? The marginalization of men in social scientific research on infertility', *Reproductive Biomedicine Online*, 27(3): 225–35.

Culley, L., Hudson, N. and Van Rooij, F. (eds) (2009) *Marginalised Reproduction: Ethnicity, Infertility and Reproductive Technologies*, London: Earthscan.

Daniels, C. (2006) *Exposing Men: The Science and Politics of Male Reproduction*, Oxford: Oxford University Press.

de Boer, M.L. (2022) 'Virile infertile men, and other representations of in/fertile hegemonic masculinity in fiction television series', in T. Jones and K. Pachucki (eds), *The COVID Pandemic: Essays, Book Reviews, and Poems*, Cham: Springer Nature Switzerland, pp 147–64.

Dermott, E. (2008) *Intimate Fatherhood: A Sociological Analysis*, London: Routledge.

Dermott, E and Miller, E. (2015) 'More than the sum of its parts? Contemporary fatherhood policy, practice and discourse', *Families, Relationships and Societies*, 4(2): 183–95.

Dolan, A., Lomas, T., Ghobara, T. and Hartshorne, G. (2017) '"It's like taking a bit of masculinity away from you": Towards a theoretical understanding of men's experiences of infertility', *Sociology of Health and Illness*, 39(6): 878–92.

Elliott, K. (2016) 'Caring masculinities: Theorizing an emerging concept', *Men and Masculinities*, 19(3): 240–59.

Foster, S., Pomerantz, A., Bell, K., Carvallo, M., Lee, J. and Lee, J. (2022) 'Victims of virility: Honor endorsement, stigma, and men's use of erectile dysfunction medication', *Psychology of Men and Masculinities*, 23(1): 47–58.

Gannon, K., Glover, L. and Abel, P. (2004) 'Masculinity, infertility, stigma and media reports', *Social Science and Medicine*, 59(6): 1169–75.

Goffman, E. (1963) *Stigma: On the Management of Spoiled Identity*, Englewood Cliffs, NJ: Prentice-Hall.

Gough, B. (2018) *Contemporary Masculinities: Embodiment, Emotion and Wellbeing*, Cham: Springer.

Hadley, R.A. (2020) 'Male broodiness: Does the desire for fatherhood affect men?', *Psychreg Journal of Psychology*, 4(3): 67–89.

Hanna, E. and Gough, B. (2015) 'Experiencing male infertility: A review of the qualitative research literature', *Sage Open*, 5(4).

Hanna, E. and Gough, B. (2016) 'Emoting infertility online: A qualitative analysis of men's forum posts', *Health*, 20(4): 363–82.

Hanna, E. and Gough, B. (2017) 'Men's accounts of infertility within their intimate partner relationships: An analysis of online forum discussions', *Journal of Reproductive and Infant Psychology*, 35(2): 150–8.

Hanna, E. and Gough, B. (2018) 'Searching for help online: An analysis of peer-to-peer posts on a male-only infertility forum', *Journal of Health Psychology*, 23(7): 917–28.

Hanna, E. and Gough, B. (2020) 'The social construction of male infertility: A qualitative questionnaire study of men with a male factor infertility diagnosis', *Sociology of Health and Illness*, 42(3): 465–80.

Hanna, E.S. and Gough, B. (2022) *(In)Fertile Male Bodies: Masculinities and Lifestyle Management in Neoliberal Times*, Bingley: Emerald Publishing Limited.

Hanna, E., Gough, B. and Hudson, N. (2018) 'Fit to father? Online accounts of lifestyle changes and help-seeking on a male infertility board', *Sociology of Health and Illness*, 40(6): 937–53.

Hansen, K.A. (2022) 'The ambiguity of "new" masculinities: Zayn Malik and disordered eating', *Celebrity Studies*, 13(3): 470–4.

Hearn, J., Nordberg, M., Andersson, K., Balkmar, D., Gottzén, L., Klinth, R. and Pringle, K. (2012) 'Hegemonic masculinity and beyond: 40 years of research in Sweden', *Men and Masculinities*, 15(1): 31–55.

Inhorn, M.C. (2003) '"The worms are weak": Male infertility and patriarchal paradoxes in Egypt', *Men and Masculinities*, 5(3): 236–56.

Inhorn, M.C. (2004) 'Middle Eastern masculinities in the age of new reproductive technologies: Male infertility and stigma in Egypt and Lebanon', *Medical Anthropology Quarterly*, 18(2): 162–82.

Inhorn, M. (2012) The *New Arab Man: Emergent Masculinities, Technologies, and Islam in the Middle East*, Princeton, NJ: Princeton University Press.

Johnson Jr, M. (2010) '"Just getting off": The inseparability of ejaculation and hegemonic masculinity', *The Journal of Men's Studies*, 18(3): 238–48.

LeBel, T.P. (2008) 'Perceptions of and responses to stigma', *Sociology Compass*, 2(2): 409–32.

Link, B.G. and Phelan, J.C. (2001) 'Conceptualizing stigma', *Annual Review of Sociology*, 27(1): 363–85.

Lohan, M (2015) 'Advancing research on men and reproduction', *International Journal of Men's Health*, 14(3): 214–32.

Lloyd, M. (1996) 'Condemned to be meaningful: Non-response in studies of men and infertility', *Sociology of Health and Illness*, 18(4): 433–54.

Manzoor, S. (2019) 'Inside the male fertility crisis', *Men's Health*, [online] 13 June, Available from: https://www.menshealth.com/uk/sex/a28005220/male-infertility/ [Accessed 7 June 2024].

McElvaine, R. (2017) 'The ancient metaphor that created modern sexism', *The Washington Post*, [online] 17 October, Available from: https://www.washingtonpost.com/outlook/2018/10/17/ancient-metaphor-that-created-modern-sexism/ [Accessed 7 June 2024].

Messerschmidt, J.W. (2019a), 'The salience of "hegemonic masculinity"', *Men and Masculinities*, 22(1): 85–91.

Messerschmidt, J.W. (2019b) 'Hidden in plain sight: On the omnipresence of hegemonic masculinities', *Masculinities: A Journal of Identity and Culture*, (12): 14–29.

Morman, M.T. and Floyd, K. (2002) 'A "changing culture of fatherhood": Effects on affectionate communication, closeness, and satisfaction in men's relationships with their fathers and their sons', *Western Journal of Communication*, 66(4): 395–411.

Remennick, L. (2000) 'Childless in the land of imperative motherhood: Stigma and coping among infertile Israeli women', *Sex Roles*, 43: 821–41.

Riessman, C.K. (2000) 'Stigma and everyday resistance practices: Childless women in South India', *Gender and Society*, 14(1): 111–35.

Rome, J.M. (2020) 'Blogging wounded manhood: Negotiating hegemonic masculinity and the crisis of the male (in)fertile body', *Women's Studies in Communication*, 44(1): 44–64.

Smith, I., Knight, T., Fletcher, R. and Macdonald, J.A. (2020) 'When men choose to be childless: An interpretative phenomenological analysis', *Journal of Social and Personal Relationships*, 37(1): 325–44.

Throsby, K. and Gill, R. (2004) '"It's different for men": Masculinity and IVF', *Men and Masculinities*, 6(4): 330–48.

Vares, T., Potts, A., Gavey, N. and Grace, V.M. (2003) 'Hard sell, soft sell: Men read Viagra ads', *Media International Australia*, 108(1): 101–14.

Whiteford, L.M. and Gonzalez, L. (1995) 'Stigma: The hidden burden of infertility', *Social Science and Medicine*, 40(1): 27–36.

5

On the Process of Becoming a Body Fascist: Stigma and Shame in the Moral Economy of Exercise

Kass Gibson

Introduction

Sociologists of health and medicine have long documented how health has become a preoccupation of daily life. As part of this process, significant shifts have occurred in how health and being healthy are understood. The most important shift, for this chapter, is Robert Crawford's (1984, 76) observation that 'health is a moral discourse, an opportunity to reaffirm shared values of a culture; a way to express what it means to be a moral person'. This chapter examines how exercise and physical activity have become central to demonstrating to yourself and others your moral standing. More specifically, I illustrate how exercise is situated within a 'moral economy' that promotes 'body fascism' (terms that I clearly define later in this introduction), and how this reflects and reinforces stigma as an embodied process. In doing so, I build on calls from Graham Scambler (2004) to develop a sociological explanation of stigma by drawing on Norbert Elias' figurational sociology.

In developing this explanation, I follow Elias' (1978) view of our bodies, relationships, and lived experiences as processes. I argue stigma is a process where the experience of feeling less powerful or less worthy than others is interpreted as individual inferiority or failing (Elias and Scotson, 1994). Viewing stigma as a process highlights not only the possibilities and potentialities for change, but also how stigma is intimately tied to processes of social (and individual) change. These possibilities are evident in the interplay between our intended actions and their unintended outcomes, shaped as they are by the mutual, but not necessarily equal, (power) relationships that make up our lives (which Elias refers to as 'figurations'). From this perspective, stigma involves the maintenance and reproduction of social boundaries and the recognition of social/self-control within figurations. Following Elias (1978), stigma is a component of figurations evident in how we seek to exhibit control over (human) nature through technological developments and change (for example, the use of fitness technologies to change our bodies), over groups of people through governmental structures and institutional processes (for example, through recommendations regarding physical activity levels or physical activity health promotion initiatives), and over our drives and desires (for example, self-control in relation to food and eating and self-discipline to 'adhere' to exercise regimes) through learned, and socially condoned, patterns of self-control. Embedded in these processes and habits are how we interpret and express a range of emotional responses (especially shame, referred to by Thomas Scheff [2004] as 'the master emotion') through individual and collective behaviours. I argue that stigma is an inherent aspect of exercise practices, given the significance of emotional experiences in and through exercise, and impression management as matters of our daily lives. As such, stigmas are created and recognised through emotional responses connected to the transgressions of social norms relating to bodies and both the known and presumed effects of physical activity on them.

Two emotional responses are key here: shame and embarrassment. Elias (2000) identifies shame as feelings related to knowing we have breached social norms, while embarrassment is felt when we believe others have breached social norms. I explore how these emotions connect to stigma as an embodied process, through what I am terming the moral economy of exercise, to refer to how health as a discourse of morality and moral judgements are produced and circulated about our bodies (including stigma) in, through, and about exercise. I use the term moral economy to highlight not only links between emotional responses (like shame) and stigma, but also how moral judgements are embedded in assumptions regarding exercise and health. My identification of a moral economy is inspired by Sara Ahmed (2004, 119), who uses the term 'affective economies' to show how emotions and emotional reactions are produced and circulated to 'align individuals with communities – or bodily space with social space – through the very intensity of their attachments'.

Rather than viewing exercise as another affective economy, I seek to show how moral judgements are produced and circulated in particular historical, social, and emotional contexts. Indeed, changing attitudes towards bodily display, gender, and sexuality, as well as the rise of individualism and body modification, can create moral ambiguity and plurality. Fewer actions and traits are accepted as morally praiseworthy in contemporary Western societies, yet the pursuit of health through fitness has become one of the few unambiguous moral goods (hence, a moral economy of exercise). Within such a context, Conrad (1994) describes 'wellness as virtue', where the praiseworthiness and social acceptability of being active are at least as important as the realisation, or otherwise, of the health benefits of activity.

The moral economy is closely connected to the concept of 'body fascism': an understanding of our bodies that views them as objects with the job of producing maximum work and minimising disease risk through being fit. This links idealised body shapes (those achieved through rigorous commitment to exercise) with notions of morally praiseworthy and responsible citizenship – put simply, through the conflation of being physically fit with being morally fit. Conflating physical and moral fitness has created a moral economy of exercise in which we all directly or indirectly trade. In this 'economy', if we are seen to be physically active, we acquire greater moral value, whereas the opposite is true for inactivity. The moral economy of exercise is the context through which stigma (as a process) plays out.

With the previously discussed underpinning ideas in mind, this chapter begins by exploring how exercise and physical activity have come to be understood as key aspects of being healthy. In doing so, I argue that despite historian of sports medicine Jack Berryman (2010, 2012) and others (Tipton, 2014) documenting how physicians and philosophers from ancient to modern times have advocated physical activity, *exercise* has been 'invented' only recently. As I demonstrate in the next section, viewing exercise as invented recently highlights how concerns with structuring and organising bodily movement as an integral component of public health and personal self- and healthcare is less about physiological or psychological impacts movement has on bodies, and more about how health has become a moral discourse. This discourse is linked to the (re-)definition of health as a complete state of wellbeing (Larsen, 2022), which can (and must) be individually achieved (through, for example, regular exercise and physical activity).

Following the section on the invention of exercise, and consistent with Elias' (2000) study of emotional restraint as a mechanism of social control, I show how shame is central to both the moral economy of exercise and stigma as an embodied process. Extending Scambler's (2004) work, I argue that shame and stigma are central to our experiences and understandings of (in)activity. Given the observed connections between shame (and embarrassment) as emotions and stigma as an embodied process, I demonstrate how being (in)active today involves navigating body fascism.

The 'invention of exercise' and a moral economy

Historian Shelly McKenzie (2013) outlines the various governmental, commercial, and scientific industries that promoted physical activity through the latter half of the 20th century. In doing so, McKenzie (2013) documents that not only were the types, intensities, and duration of different activities debated (debates that are still ongoing), but also that the necessity and even efficacy of being active were subject to debate. In stark contrast to contemporary concerns focused on the negative impact of inactivity, public health reformers through the late 19th and early 20th century were concerned with the negative impact of overexertion (especially for women [Chisholm, 2005]). Indeed, the findings of a 1957 review of medical literature by physician Donald Dukelow now seems unthinkable. Dukelow concluded that, despite hundreds of published papers on the topic, researchers were unable to say whether being active was 'beneficial, harmful, or of no consequence' (Dukelow, 1957, 24). McKenzie (2013) argues that the shift in attitudes – sociologically, scientifically, and politically – to physical activity from a poorly evidenced, socially undesirable, and dubious endeavour to the 'best buy in public health' and a 'miracle cure' (Academy of Medical Royal Colleges, 2015) constitutes a process of the 'invention of exercise' (McKenzie, 2013, 2).

To say exercise was invented only in the last 80 or so years does not contradict, for example, the ancient Indian physician and 'father of surgery', Susruta, 'prescribing' movement over two-and-a-half thousand years ago (Tipton, 2014). Rather, it shows how attitudes towards physical activity and movement reflect cultural norms and standards of behaviour. Put differently, conceptualising physical activity as exercise speaks not only to how activity is structured (for example, through guidelines for intensity of activity, or via particular systems of movement, like aerobics or CrossFit), but the attitudes and values evident in, and used to explain and justify, being active. For example, changes regarding the appropriateness of exercising (for example, being sweaty or flushed) and different understandings of desirable body shapes have influenced the advocacy and uptake of exercise (McKenzie, 2013). Attitudes towards exercise practices and ideas about fitness are shaped by cultural beliefs and morality, such as attitudes towards sexuality and gender. This underlines how exercise is shaped by the various meanings attached to it, rather than anything inherent to the physical or physiological adaptations that arise from movement *per se*.

Exercise was invented in a particular context of post-war affluence, in North America particularly, where physical needs (for example, access to enough (safe) food, secure and warm housing, and clean drinking water) were addressed for large swathes of society – though primarily the middle classes – on an unprecedented scale. However, the abundance of food, widespread accessibility of mechanised transportation, dynamic changes in values towards sexuality, rising availability of effective medications, and increasingly sophisticated and successful medical interventions created new definitions of health (Larsen, 2022) and associated health concerns. These new concerns (for example, cardiac disease and diabetes) became evident – or invented – as other concerns were increasingly controlled (Gibson and Malcolm, 2020). Exercise, then, was invented at a time when health was being established as a moral discourse, with gluttony and idleness making stark comebacks as objects of moral concern. Therefore, exercising to be healthy was a way to demonstrate contemporary notions of character, identity, and responsible citizenship (Crawford, 1984) – in short, exercising evidences your worth in the moral economy of exercise.

Indeed, Peter Conrad (1994, 398) identified that 'the body provides a forum for moral discourse, and wellness-seeking becomes a vehicle for setting oneself among the righteous'. Similarly, Nichter and Nichter (1991) described getting into shape (that is, seeking a morally praiseworthy body shape) as a morality play. The moral economy of exercise shapes our expectations and experiences to the extent that we feel good after/from exercise because we feel that we should – or, perhaps, having achieved what is culturally framed as an unambiguous moral good, we feel we deserve to. As such, the conflation of morality, emotional experience, and physicality extends Ahmed's (2004) affective economies into moral economies. The invention of exercise, then, is tied to the development of a moral discourse related to changes in how health is conceptualised, politicised, and experienced. Beliefs that you should take responsibility for your health through being physically active required a definitional shift from clinical definitions of health as the absence of disease, to health as a state of complete physical, mental, and social wellbeing (Larsen, 2022). When health is more than not being ill, fitness becomes a proxy for health.

Where fitness has been viewed as a proxy for public health, exercise cultures have longstanding and inglorious links with biological management and belonging, including eugenics and fascism (Zweiniger-Bargielowska, 2010). For example, 'muscular Christianity' in Victorian Britain valued muscular (male) bodies as evidence of strong individual morals as well as legitimised colonial activities, imperialism, and racial purity (Hall, 1994). Such notions continue to connect muscular corporeality to the contemporary far-right and associated militaristic, nationalistic, White supremacist, and misogynistic philosophies (Wolley and Luger, 2023). Questions of responsible citizenship and belonging circulating in the moral economy of exercise become evident in questions of access to welfare institutions generally and healthcare institutions specifically (Meloni, 2016). Roberta Bivans (2015) highlighted how the National Health Service in the UK, through the assessment, treatment, and management of our bodies, has made health and healthcare important sites for negotiating citizenship and belonging in legal, policy, and cultural terms. In the next section, I build on Scambler's (2004) call for a sociological theorising of stigma to show how stigma (in the moral economy of exercise) is an embodied process.

Understanding stigma as an embodied process

Scambler's (2004) re-evaluation of stigma highlights the relationship between shame and stigma. Scambler reflects on 'felt stigma' to describe the shame associated with being reduced to a condition, and the fear of encountering 'enacted stigma', which is the act of shaming. Others have also worked to articulate the relationship between shame and stigma. For example: Walker (2014, 50) states 'shame and stigma are intricately connected to the point whereby they can be treated as being almost synonymous'; Stunkel and Wong (2012, 52) identify, historically, that 'shame and guilt were used to describe a stigma – a perceived difference between a behaviour or an attribute or an ideal standard'; and Goffman (1953, 18) claims 'shame becomes a central possibility' when perceived points of difference are apparent.

At their core, these analyses interpret stigma as disruptions in not only what we may be able to do, but also how we feel about, and see, ourselves and our futures. In the moral economy of exercise, (the avoidance of) stigma and shame shape motivations for why we are active. This may be to achieve a desirable body shape to mould how we feel about and see ourselves, or to be healthy as an investment in our future. Scambler (2004) highlights how his initial formulations and analyses of shame and stigma (as largely representative of the medical sociology field more broadly) failed to address how large-scale issues, such as social organisation, social change, and power, reflect and reinforce stigma as well as uncritically accept the epistemic authority of biomedicine. Indeed, Luna Dolezal (2022) demonstrates the need for healthcare professionals to be aware of how their actions, manifest through positions of social power, can be biographically disruptive for people and how shame, perceived or realised, enacted or felt, shapes clinical interactions.

While I share Scambler's (2004) desire to build a sociological understanding of stigma – that explores the relationship between shame and stigma and their connection to broader sociocultural, political, and bodily processes – I believe Scambler's approach remains limited in how far it can account for how individuals' attitudes, behaviours, and activities (including those related to our bodies, health, and exercise) are products of a number of mutual, but not necessarily equal, relationships (within figurations). Scambler (2004, 40, emphasis in original) starts to make this point:

> Sociological acknowledgement is required too of a logic of shame that requires/orders/establishes the parameters for *relations of stigma* that might be studied in *figurations* ranging from the micro-world of the individual household or office to the macro-worlds of global exchange. Such a logic of shame might in different *figurations* issue in relations of stigma … There is potential here for a more comprehensive sociological appreciation and explanation of stigma, felt and enacted, which extends beyond traditional interactionist agendas to encompass a full range of structural antecedents *and their interrelations* across numerous and varied figurations.

Scambler's later work (Scambler, 2018) evaluates structural antecedents and relations of stigma, particularly class in financial capitalism, revealing the weaponisation of stigma manifest in welfare reduction, blaming individuals for their poverty, the rise of populist politics, and populist political leaders' successful demonisation of marginalised groups. What is peculiar about both Scambler's initial call and later work is the lack of engagement with figurations as a specific sociological concept. This is surprising given Scambler's awareness of figurations and figurational sociology (which is a name given to the school of thought based on Elias' ideas). Later in this chapter, I aim to show how figurational sociology can be useful in understanding both stigma more broadly as well as in the moral economy of exercise specifically.

Viewing stigma as a process emphasises the interplay between planned/intended actions and unplanned/unintended outcomes due to the various interdependent relationships through which we live our lives. Emphasising how our lives are constituted by connections between ourselves, our bodies, other people, ideas, and things (that is, in figurations) emphasises how people can and must learn and internalise, often without realising, socially sanctioned ideas about how our bodies should look, function, and feel into taken-for-granted ideas, actions, and emotional experiences. Elias (2002, 214) explains: 'Since people are more or less dependent on each other, first by nature and then by social learning, through education, socialisation, and socially generated reciprocal needs, they exist, one might venture to say, only as pluralities, only in figurations'.

My identification of Scambler's failure to engage more fully with theorising the implications of studying the 'structural antecedents' and 'relations of deviance' (see Scambler, 2004) of stigma implicit in (different) figurations as a specific concept is not a *gotcha* among sociologists policing the use of sociological theory. My critique of Scambler's re-evaluation of stigma (both felt and enacted) is that he fails to account for the importance of emotional restraint and embedded moral evaluations as dominant social control mechanisms (that is, discipline via self-surveillance) within figurations *and* concomitantly the varying embodied experiences of bodies in and through exercise (Gibson and Malcolm, 2020). Scambler fails to address how deeply embodied stigma is; stigma is neither simply moralistic discourse (for example, messages about how you *should* be exercising) nor prejudice (for example, towards certain body shapes or abilities). Stigma is felt *deeply*. Stigma is embodied (or corp*oreal*) and, as such, is more than a reflective, cognitive process. Stigma manifests in the evaluation of bodies (our own and others') as a meter of good citizenship. Our (in)activity is a barometer of our individual emotional regulation and self-control, social relationships shaping ideas of health, beauty, and desire, and long-term historical processes, such as the invention of exercise. Despite calling to understand stigma within figurations, Scambler (2004, 2018) fails to fully engage with what sits at the heart of figurational sociology: namely, processes of social, and then internal, personal self-regulation reflective of shifting social relationships (figurations). Elias' identification of the significance of feelings of disgust, shame, and embarrassment towards specific social practices helps explain this further.

For Elias (2000, 2002), shame is the feeling of anxiety due to the transgression of social norms, while embarrassment is the perception that *others* have transgressed social norms. As outlined earlier, shame is an embodied process. Central to Elias' scholarship is understanding how shifting cultural orientations towards our bodies manifest in both our experiences and knowledge of our bodies. For example, Oli Williams and Ellen Annandale (2020) explore this in relation to weight-related stigma. They highlight how people use physical activity to cope with stigma associated with them being 'overweight'. In particular, they show how stigma is deeply felt (embodied) not only because of the emotions generated (which they describe as psychosomatic stress and also 'carnal cues'), but also precisely on account of moralised views of physical activity and exercise replete with assumptions of (ir)responsibility. As such, when weight gain is assumed to be the product of insufficient amounts of exercise (poor self-discipline) and eating too much (poor self-control), people would still use physical activity and exercise to reconcile how their bodies looked with the exercise they would engage in.

Put differently, the experience of exercise (physical exertion, sweating, flushness, aching muscles) helped the people in the study to counteract the characterisation of them as both physically and morally unfit. In short, it helped them to feel better about themselves. This is one way that the process of stigmatisation occurs through the moral economy of exercise as an embodied process. It informs and influences how we perceive bodies and shapes our emotions to the extent that we derive satisfaction from physical activity not just because of the presumed health benefits, but because being active aligns with culturally ingrained notions of moral excellence. Consequently, the sense of accomplishment and deservingness described by those in Williams and Annandale's (2020) study stems not only from the physiological effects of exercise, but also from fulfilling what society deems as a clear moral imperative even (or perhaps especially) when idealised body shapes are not evident.

Elias (2002) describes and analyses how people learn and internalise (often without realising) social norms about how our bodies should look, function, and feel. This process manifests into taken-for-granted habits (for example, how we dress, eat, and exercise) that are informed by the way exercise has been invented. Philosopher Martha Nussbaum (2005, 272) highlights the power of shame as:

> A productive and potentially creative emotion. Shame is subtle, for it goads us onwards with regard to many different types of goals and

ideals, some of them valuable. In that sense, it is not inherently self-deceptive, nor does it always express a desire to be a sort of being one is not. It often tells us the truth: certain goals are valuable, and we have failed to live up to them.

Elias (2000) identifies how what is shameful and embarrassing changes over time to reflect changing social norms and cultural values. Elias (2000) focuses particularly on how behaviours and attitudes once considered acceptable become increasingly shameful or repugnant as social norms evolve as *advancing thresholds of shame*. Changing thresholds of shame are powerful aspects of social control. As people seek to avoid the psychosomatic stress of feeling shame or being embarrassed, these actions are reinforced, since avoiding those behaviours demonstrates the self-control and self-restraint that defines moral praiseworthiness and responsible citizenship.

Both Deborah Lupton (1995) and Chris Shilling (2013) have taken Elias' (2000) insights on shame, embarrassment, and social control to develop the idea of the 'civilized body'. Shilling (2013, 156) highlights how our bodies become sites where codes of behaviour are located and expressed, which contributes to the possibilities for 'differentiating between individuals on the basis of their bodily worth'. The ways exercise shapes bodies, then, are taken as indicative of both identity and moral worth, as active lifestyles become synonymous with being a 'good' citizen. For example, Mirjam Stuij (2011, 797) shows how differentiated patterns in trends in body weight between social groups, and the 'slenderness code', demonstrates how particular body shapes embody historically and culturally specific values. Within the so-called 'obesogenic environments' of contemporary developed nations, slender bodies are valued as markers of self-control.

Likewise, Louise Mansfield (2010) highlights how the longstanding cultural revulsion of body fat is reinforced in sport and exercise cultures, which subsequently reinforces middle-class habits, values, and behaviours. In the moral economy of exercise, good citizens are understood as making a 'net contribution' to society as their health status is considered not to be a drain on health services (or the public purse more broadly). Stigmatisation, then, takes place when people are viewed as (un)able to conform with hallmarks of being 'tightly contained, consciously managed, subject to continual self-surveillance' (Lupton, 1995, 22) as healthy, attractive, and *good* citizens.

Elias (1978) also evidenced how enhanced susceptibility to shame and embarrassment, contoured by social status, are actively fostered as a component of efforts at behaviour change. Shame and stigma are central components of attitudes towards being active. Recalling Elias' differentiation between shame and embarrassment, many of us feel shame about our bodies when we recognise them as not evidencing morally praiseworthy behaviours. We can also feel embarrassed when we recognise that in others. We are embarrassed for them and/or concerned about how others will act towards them because of what we know their body/perceived inactivity is taken to represent. As such, within the moral economy of exercise, the civilised body is simultaneously a marker against which 'uncivilised' bodies are stigmatised and shamed, *and* a defence against shame for those who are considered to take this morally praiseworthy form.

That being said, stigma, shame, and exercise are not just issues of perception or cultural values. Being physically (in)active does influence health and wellbeing outcomes. And avoiding shame and stigma can motivate people to be active, which may result in positive health outcomes for them. However, stigma is associated with failure to meet valued norms *and* inextricably linked to negative health outcomes at the population level. Peter Freund (2015, 151), from a figurational perspective, has shown that 'social locations or positions in such figurations may vary by gender, socio-economic, racial, ethnic, and cultural status. Socio-cultural inequalities in social figurations and structures have been linked to health inequalities'. Consequently, shame circulates as we blame ourselves (or are blamed by others) for not being active enough. This is because, as the risk of life-threatening, acute illness reduces, the more rational and normal it seems to invest time and money into proactively preserving our health through exercise, as well as the denial of our impulses. Stigma is attached to those who are viewed as *deserving* of their ill-health through their failure to be rational – for their failure to take personal responsibility by, for example, exercising regularly.

Freund (2015) extends this point by demonstrating how Elias develops Erving Goffman's emphasis on the 'dramaturgical self' (which highlights the various strategies people use to present themselves in a favourable light to others) as an embodied process central to understanding stigma. Taking Elias' broader point about how drives and desires are interwoven into the fabric of social history, we can understand how stigma is experienced and (re)produced in, through, and about exercise and health because it entails (a commitment to) altering our bodily functioning and composition. To understand shame and stigma, we must address how emotional responses regulate our behaviours in accordance with social norms and expectations. As I have noted, shame and embarrassment are significant, indeed central, components of social control (Binkley, 2009). From such a perspective, Elias prefigures Scambler's (2004) critique of sociologists reducing stigma to biography:

> At present the tendency is to discuss the problem of social stigmatisation as if it were simply a question of people showing individually a pronounced dislike of other people as individuals. A well-known way of conceptualising such an observation is to classify it as prejudice. However, that means perceiving only at the individual level something

which cannot be understood without perceiving it at the same time at the group level. (Elias and Scotson, 1994, xx)

Most sociologists studying stigma acknowledge that to 'perceive' stigma at the 'group' level requires addressing issues of power. For Elias (Elias and Scotson, 1994, xx), 'the ability of one group to pin a badge of human inferiority on another group and to make it stick was a function of a specific figuration'. The ability to make stigma 'stick' is intimately tied to shifting and developing emotional responses – put differently, an embodied process. In the next section, I introduce the idea of body fascism to explain the ideas that shape collective thinking (psychogenesis) that has crystallised the moral economy of exercise, stigma, and shame as cultural norms in physical activity.

Body fascism, stigma, and the moral economy of exercise

Body fascism is usually used as a term to describe discriminatory views based on appearance and/or weight (Griffin, 2017). However, within the moral economy of exercise, body fascism is more complicated, and prevalent, than discriminatory views. Many critiques demonstrate how attractiveness, fitness, health, and wellbeing are assumed to be synonymous with narrowly defined idealised body shapes (civilised bodies). Body fascism highlights how this assumption marks certain body shapes as (ir)responsible and (un)attractive (or uncivilised). As such, body fascism is directed at all bodies, not just those deemed unhealthy. Body fascism is a deep-seated ideological framing of our bodies that makes the connection of idealised body shapes (that is, those achieved through rigorous commitment to exercise), and notions of responsible citizenship seem self-evident and obvious. In other words, body fascism underpins taken-for-granted assumptions that exercise is an unambiguous moral good. I maintain that body fascism is useful for understanding stigma and shame in exercise cultures by highlighting how the processes of social control and internal self-regulation within figurations provides the glue that makes stigma stick. To better understand this, I expand body fascism beyond discriminatory views by reviewing its scholarly history.

Jean-Marie Brohm (1978) theorised body fascism as a key component of elite sport. Brohm's contemporaries critiqued how States used athletes and sport as a form of propaganda. Hitler's attempt to use the Olympic Games in 1936 to promote his government and ideals of racial superiority (although this was blown to pieces by Black American athlete Jesse Owens) is an obvious example. Brohm furthered these critiques by articulating how the political ideologies of fascism – autocracy, militarism, forcible suppression of opposition, and championing of the nation and race – manifest in sport were inscribed on the bodies of athletes, regardless of the political systems and nations from which the athletes came:

> To give some idea of the alienation involved in sport, stemming from the oppression of the body pushed to the limits of physical effort, mention still has to be made of the repression which the athletes voluntarily undergo ... The intensive practice of sport is an institutionalised celebration of the mortification of the flesh, the acting out of a sado-masochistic ideology. Its compulsive repetitiveness and sexual frustration are sure signs of the neurotic obsession of the ascetic with discipline and self-mastery. (Brohm, 1978, 23)

While sport, exercise, and physical activity are distinct (Caspersen et al, 1985), sport has historically been the most popular form of physical activity (Gibson and Malcolm, 2020). Ivan Waddington demonstrates how the invention of exercise and its positioning as an important healthcare practice has led to sporting organisations working hard to present sport not as its own cultural practice with questionable claims to the promotion of health, but as a form of exercise and means of promoting health. Evidence of this success can be seen in exercise marketing and physical activity health promotion, which (re)affirms – using Brohm's terms – the 'neurotic obsession of the ascetic with discipline and self-mastery' (psychogenesis) and 'institutionalised celebration of the mortification of the flesh' (sociogenesis).

Consider, for example, the pervasive 'no pain, no gain' mantra as well as company slogans including 'impossible is nothing' and 'just do it'. Similarly, 'This Girl Can', an exercise promotion campaign developed by Sport England to increase women's physical activity levels, championed 'sweating like a pig, feeling like a fox'. For Brohm, the core of body fascism is not the blood, sweat, and tears of exertion or winning medals and championships, but the instrumental view of our bodies as machines with the job of producing the maximum work and energy. Brian Pronger (2002) also explores how exercise instrumentalises our bodies. Pronger addresses how discourses regarding sports and exercise science (the fields of study that seek to apply 'scientific' principles to sport and exercise and endlessly debate the best forms of exercise) impose limits on how we understand being active specifically and value our bodies more generally. Stigma, then, sticks to 'undesirable' or 'unhealthy' bodies through taken-for-granted ideological framings about maximising the potential of our bodies (being fitter) as a sensible, logical, and reasonable purpose for moving.

Brohm claims that body fascism is obvious in fascist political systems but is not limited to them. Equally, body fascism is consistent regardless of contemporary and varied exercise fashions and fads (namely, debates regarding intensity of activity or which exercise style is best). The realisation of any physical changes in our individual body shapes, or broader social debates about what healthy bodies are, are less important than the consistent ideological framing of our bodies (maximising utility and minimising risk) and shifting power imbalances and interdependences.

This framing is perpetuated by the creation of an army of experts and technicians. Elsewhere, Oli Williams and I (Williams and Gibson, 2018) defined these people as 'movement intellectuals', whose work on the 'act of moving' is simultaneously an advancement of a body fascism. Examples of movement intellectuals include people such as Joe Wicks, Davina McCall, David Goggins, and Tim Noakes. Movement intellectualism, then, creates a situation where advocacy for movement is a product of political commitment (what is called body fascism) as much as the evidence base linking activity to the promotion of health. As such, movement intellectuals limit critical questioning of exercise (despite consensus being less conclusive than evidence suggests; see Gard, 2011; Piggin and Bairner, 2016), underplay and/or omit opportunity costs of exercise such as injuries (Malcolm, 2017), and claim that exercise positively influences virtues which are unknowable and unproveable (Gibson, 2023).

Perhaps the most powerful examples of this comes from Waddington (2000), who identified how the evidence base for health promotion in sport is on shaky ground. Indeed, sport is often harmful to health due to injuries, yet policy responses and initiatives fail to differentiate between exercise and sport and ignore the human aspect of these activities. As a result, the high incidence of sports injuries (30 million per year in the UK, 10 million of which are potentially serious) is often overlooked. Movement intellectuals' failure to acknowledge the opportunity costs of activity, or that being active can be anything other than a simple and obvious investment in your own health, frame exercise behaviours and body shapes where morality, praiseworthiness, and social acceptability (that is, the moral economy) of exercise are at least as important as any 'real' psychological or physical benefits. Movement intellectuals, then, are more than happy to inflate the value of exercise within the moral economy of exercise. As such, body fascism trades simultaneously on the relationship of health and fitness being positive, redoubtable, and stable, all the while vociferously debating the merits of different diets and workout plans. Indeed, the most well-known and well-used measures of success – for example, BMI (body mass index) as a measure of health and taking 10,000 steps a day as a healthcare practice – are the products of actuaries and marketing agencies, respectively. Neither are supported by robust evidence. Their ubiquity, and how we embody them through both our actions and our emotional responses to these figures, reflects Elias' identification of processed sociogenic and psychogenic changes. For example, people now commonly wear tracking technologies (for example, watches with GPS) that provide them with an approximate (though usually interpreted as an exact) daily step count, and viewing this figure can and does influence the behaviour and mood of the wearer.

Interestingly, despite the overwhelming evidence showing regular physical activity has positive impacts on overall psychological and physiological functioning and decreasing risk of ill-health, the multitudinous responses to physical activity mean specific causes and mechanisms explaining these outcomes are not particularly well understood. Obviously, there are exceptions in relation to cardiovascular functioning because of changes in mechanical efficiency of heart function, for example. However, overall, the exact mechanisms causing risk factor reduction are not especially well understood. Issues regarding hormone regulation, inhibition of certain growth factors, changes in overall caloric expenditure, and favourably altering body composition are all factors that appear to be at play. This lack of consensus is seldom evident in everyday discourse, or the value judgements of the '(un)civilised' body. Rather, debates around optimal frequency and forms of exercise abound. All the while, these debates seek to show how 'easy' and 'cheap' being active can be. These narratives are frequently used to conveniently ignore other aspects of life, society, and culture that have far more profound impacts on our health that we either have less control over, or exercise will not offset. Most obvious is health inequalities: you cannot jog your way out of poverty, nor press-up depression away. The moral economy of exercise, in which entrepreneurial movement intellectuals thrive, creates an environment ready-made for the active production, circulation, and valorisation of body fascism. Taken together, we can understand the moral economy of exercise as a process of stigmatisation whereby shame is negotiated through an embodied relationship with physical activity.

Conclusion

Positioning stigma as an embodied process requires understanding the interplay between social experiences and socially generated emotions. Exercise, then, is not simply a common-sense activity that is good for us, but rather is situated in a moral economy that symbolises recognition and enaction of a socially 'policed' moral duty and political responsibility for attaining, or maximising, health. In Eliasian terms, the moral economy of exercise is a figuration through which we understand and experience bodies – our own and those of others. So, even if we may actively resist becoming a body fascist, we must inevitably navigate body fascism in our daily lives. In many contemporary cultures, the moral economy of exercise provides taken-for-granted assumptions about bodies and physical activity that perpetually position us all in relation to a stigma. This perhaps gives new meaning to the adage 'you can run but you cannot hide'.

Stigma and shame are as much a part of exercise as sweating and raised heart rates. Said differently, physical, social, and emotional experiences must be understood in conjunction. As such, I have highlighted how previous scholarship on stigma has consistently underplayed how the physicality of exercise and emotion is entwined with social and cultural processes. As such, being active is not just about being healthy, but realising a moral achievement purchased through our labour that enhances our potential to live a prolonged life (relative to other humans). It plays on our fears of mortality and places stigma at the heart of exercise, meaning simple attitudinal shifts (either from those 'affected' or those 'perpetuating' shame and stigma) are seen as enough to address, accommodate, and overcome stigma. This promotes an individualised perspective of our emotional processes and understanding of morals, which reinforces individual responsibility for health.

Could things be different?

- Physical activity is often limited by being framed primarily as a means through which to promote health, improve productivity, and/or achieve physical attractiveness. We must reject narrow metrics of performance (for example, steps taken or weight lost) to recognise how exercise motives can extend beyond health, and seek to encourage movement pursued outside the norms that have been shaped by the moral economy of exercise.
- While shame can be motivating for some, it can be inhibitory for others. Emphasising the importance of enjoyment and sociability in exercise, sport, and physical activity may offer a more positive motivator than approaches that (however inadvertently) embed shame and stigma.

References

Academy of Medical Royal Colleges (2015) *Exercise: The Miracle Cure and the Role of the Doctor in Promoting It,* London: Academy of Medical Royal Colleges.

Ahmed, S. (2004) 'Affective economies', *Social Text,* 22(2): 117–39.

Berryman, J.W. (2010) 'Exercise is medicine: A historical perspective', *Current Sports Medicine Reports,* 9(4): 195–201.

Berryman, J.W. (2012) 'Motion and rest: Galen on exercise and health', *The Lancet,* 380: 210–11.

Binkley, S. (2009) 'The civilizing brand', *European Journal of Cultural Studies,* 12(1): 21–39.

Bivans, R. (2015) *Contagious Communities: Medicine, Migration, and the NHS in Post War Britain,* Oxford: Oxford University Press.

Brohm, J. (1978) *Sport: A Prison of Measured Time,* London: Ink Links Ltd.

Caspersen C.J., Powell K.E. and Christenson G.M. (1985) 'Physical activity, exercise, and physical fitness: Definitions and distinctions for health-related research', *Public Health Reports,* 100(2): 126–31.

Chisholm, A. (2005) 'Incarnations and practices of feminine rectitude: Nineteenth-century gymnastics for U.S. women', *Journal of Social History,* 38(3): 737–63.

Conrad, P. (1994) 'Wellness as virtue: Morality and the pursuit of health', *Culture, Medicine and Psychiatry,* 18: 385–401.

Crawford, R. (1984) 'A cultural account of "health": Control, release, and the social body', in J. McKinlay (ed), *Issues in the Political Economy of Health Care,* London: Tavistock, pp 61–103.

Dolezal, L. (2022) 'Shame anxiety, stigma and clinical encounters', *Journal of Evaluation in Clinical Practice,* 28(5): 854–60.

Dukelow, D.A. (1957) 'A doctor looks at exercise and fitness', *Journal of Health, Physical Education, Recreation,* 28(6): 24–67.

Elias, N. (1978) *What is Sociology?,* London: Hutchinson.

Elias, N. (2000) *The Civilizing Process,* Oxford: Blackwell Publishers.

Elias, N. (2002) *The Society of Individuals,* Oxford: Blackwell Publishers.

Elias, N. and Scotson, J. (1994) *The Established and the Outsiders* (2nd edn), London: Sage.

Freund, P. (2015) 'Norbert Elias and Erving Goffman: Civilised-dramaturgical bodies, social status and health inequalities', in F. Collyer (ed), *The Palgrave Handbook of Social Theory in Health, Illness and Medicine,* London: Palgrave Macmillan, pp 158–73.

Gard, M. (2011) *The End of the Obesity Epidemic,* London: Routledge.

Gibson, K. (2023) 'Information hazards and moral harm: Sport and exercise science laboratories as sites of moral catastrophes', in J. Cherrington and J. Black (eds), *Sport and Physical Activity in Catastrophic Environments,* London: Routledge, pp 177–92.

Gibson, K. and Malcolm, D. (2020) 'Theorizing physical activity health promotion: Towards an Eliasian framework for the analysis of health and medicine', *Social Theory & Health,* 18: 66–85.

Griffin, G. (2017) *A Dictionary of Gender Studies,* Oxford University Press.

Goffman, E. (1953) *Stigma: Notes on the Management of Spoiled Identity,* London: Penguin Books.

Hall, D.E. (ed) (1994) *Muscular Christianity: Embodying the Victorian Age,* Cambridge: Cambridge University Press.

Larsen, L.T. (2022) 'Not merely the absence of disease: A genealogy of the WHO's positive health definition', *History of the Human Sciences,* 35(1): 111–31.

Lupton, D. (1995) *The Imperative of Health: Public Health and the Regulated Body,* London: Sage.

Malcolm, D. (2017) *Sport, Medicine and Health: The Medicalization of Sport?*, London: Routledge.

Mansfield, L. (2010) 'Fit, fat and feminine? The stigmatization of fat women in fitness gyms', in E. Kennedy and P. Markula (eds), *Women and Exercise: The Body, Health and Consumerism,* London: Routledge, pp 81–101.

McKenzie, S. (2013) *Getting Physical: The Rise of Fitness Culture in America,* Lawrence, KS: University Press of Kansas.

Meloni, M. (2016) *Political Biology: Science and Social Values in Human Heredity from Eugenics to Epigenetics,* London: Palgrave Macmillan.

Nichter, M. and Nichter, M. (1991) 'Hype and weight', *Medical Anthropology,* 13(3): 249–84.

Nussbaum, M. (2005) 'Inscribing the face: Shame, stigma, and punishment', in S. Macedo and M.S. Williams (eds), *Political Exclusion and Domination,* New York: New York University Press, pp 259–302.

Piggin, J. and Bairner, A. (2016) 'The global physical inactivity pandemic: An analysis of knowledge production', *Sport, Education, and Society,* 21(2): 131–47.

Pronger, B. (2002) *Body Fascism: Salvation in the Technology of Physical Fitness,* Toronto: University of Toronto Press.

Scambler, G. (2004) 'Re-framing stigma: Felt and enacted stigma and challenges to the sociology of chronic and disabling conditions', *Social Theory and Health,* 2: 29–46.

Scambler, G. (2018) 'Heaping blame on shame: "Weaponising stigma" for neoliberal times', *The Sociological Review,* 66(4): 766–82.

Scheff, T.J. (2004) 'Elias, Freud and Goffman: Shame as the master emotion', in S. Loyal and S. Quilley (eds), *The Sociology of Norbert Elias,* Cambridge: Cambridge University Press, pp 229–44.

Shilling, C. (2013) *The Body and Social Theory* (3rd edn), London: Sage.

Stuij, M. (2011) 'Explaining trends in body weight: Offer's rational and myopic choice vs Elias' theory of civilizing processes', *Social History of Medicine,* 24(3): 796–812.

Stunkel, D. and Wong, V. (2012) 'Stigma', in I.M. Lubkin and P.D. Larsen (eds), *Chronic Illness: Impact and Intervention,* Burlington, MA: Jones and Bartlett, pp 47–74.

Tipton, C.M. (ed) (2014) *History of Exercise Physiology,* Champagne, IL: Human Kinetics.

Waddington, I. (2000) 'Sport and health', in J. Coakley and E. Dunning (eds), *Handbook of Sports Studies,* London: Sage, pp 405–59.

Walker, R. (2014) *The Shame of Poverty,* Oxford: Oxford University Press.

Williams, O. and Annandale, E. (2020) 'Obesity, stigma and reflexive embodiment', *Health,* 24(4): 421–41.

Williams, O. and Gibson, K. (2018) 'Exercise as a poisoned elixir: Inactivity, inequality and intervention', *Qualitative Research in Sport, Exercise and Health*, 10(4): 412–28.

Woolley, D. and Luger, J. (2023) 'The deviant leisure of gym bodies, militarized branding and fascistic creeps', in I.R. Lamond and R. Garland (eds), *Deviant Leisure and Events of Deviance: A Transgressive Compendium*, Cham: Springer International Publishing, pp 143–172.

Zweiniger-Bargielowska, I. (2010) *Managing the Body: Beauty, Health, and Fitness in Britain 1880–1939*, Oxford: Oxford University Press.

6

Recalibrating Anti-Stigma: Avoiding Binary Thinking and 'Destigmatisation Drift' in Public Health

Oli Williams, Amy Chandler, Gareth M. Thomas, and Tanisha Spratt

Introduction

How stigma should be approached by public health agencies is a divisive issue. Within public health, stigma is framed as both a solution (that protects people's health) and a problem (that damages people's health). Public health agencies, in turn, deploy stigma as a strategy in some settings *and* campaign to remove it in others. This twin approach is loaded with tensions and complexities that receive insufficient critical attention. Instead, the issue is frequently reduced to pro-/anti-stigma lobbying. This binary logic serves for or against arguments but undermines attempts to understand and address stigma.

In this chapter, we problematise the pro-/anti-stigma binary to highlight the need to recalibrate the theory and practice of 'anti-stigma'. We begin by outlining how sociological theorisation helps move analyses of stigma away from the lure of simplification and, instead, offers a vehicle for interrogating how and why the social production of stigma unevenly disadvantages people throughout society. From there, we identify how the moral certainty of pro-/anti-stigma lobbies obstructs acknowledgement and understanding of the complexity, inconsistency, and diversity of stigma and its effects. We continue this critique by focusing on anti-stigma efforts in the field of mental health. We propose a novel concept – 'destigmatisation drift' – to explain how approaches to anti-stigma can paradoxically undermine efforts to address the social drivers of suffering, illness, and stigma. Finally, we explore tensions in anti-stigma theory and practice through the examples of 'obesity', anorexia, and self-harm. Each case demonstrates that the moral and practical considerations of addressing stigma are far from straightforward, and why pro-/anti-stigma framing is an inadequate route to understanding or addressing these issues.

When referring to stigma in this chapter, we are describing a social process whereby a person or group are negatively characterised because they transgress a social norm or standard and, consequently, are expected to navigate shame. This attends to Goffman's (1963, 3) conceptualisation of stigma as 'an attribute that is deeply discrediting' and as something that plays out in interactions between people. It also recognises that stigma is part of a political economy, where powerful actors/institutions 'activate' stigma to their benefit (Tyler and Slater, 2018, 732). As such, we find Scambler's (2018) 'weaponisation of stigma' concept particularly instructive. Scambler (2018) asserts that, because many societies are increasingly governed through a heightened focus on individualisation and personal responsibility, stigma (norms marking personal deficiency, non-conformance, or shame) can be redefined as deviance (norms marking moral deficit, non-compliance, or blame). This implies a distinction between stigma/shame and deviance/blame that we endorse. For Scambler (2018, 771), stigma 'might usefully be regarded as an offence against norms of shame, while deviance might be seen as an offence against norms of blame'. For us, the coupling of stigma/shame and deviance/blame, to actively 'weaponise' stigma against certain people, should be a central concern of stigma analyses. Analyses of stigma are incomplete without considering not only how shame impacts peoples' lives, but also how and why a person or group has been stigmatised. Particular concerns for us are:

- How and why does stigma disadvantage some people more than others?
- Who has the power to stigmatise, and how do they benefit from this?
- How and why has stigmatisation been operationalised? Has it been weaponised to assert fault or (ir)responsibility?
- What is the impact of stigma at a micro-level (how it affects peoples' everyday lives) and macro-level (how it contributes to the creation and entrenchment of inequalities, marginalisation, and suffering)?

In our respective research, we engage with these concerns as they relate to health/illness and medicine/public health. This chapter considers how the pro-/anti-stigma binary intersects with, and can impede, these lines of inquiry.

Pro-/anti-stigma lobbies: increased certainty, reduced understanding?

Brewis and Wutich (2019) outline a divisive reality between disciplines in the field of global health: stigma is viewed as both a problem requiring solutions *and* a solution to problems. This tension will be familiar to those working across public health. Many respond by adopting a pro- or anti-stigma position. Brewis and Wutich (2019, 11) claim 'between these two views lies the unchartered territory that must be navigated to create truly just, sustainable health'. This position goes against the either/or reasoning that tends to characterise entrenched pro-/anti-stigma positions. What is inhibiting exploration of the complexity between them?

In his commentary on the ethics of using stigma in public health, Bayer (2008) considers shifting public opinion over time. Stigma was commonplace in the 19th century, with the rise of public health as a profession, before the HIV/AIDS pandemic of the 1980s/1990s demonstrated how it can heighten the vulnerability of affected groups and impede attempts to treat and control disease. Despite this, Bayer (2008) shows, through the example of smoking, that in the 20th and 21st centuries, stigma once again became a common public health strategy. Bayer (2008, 467) argues that this was made possible by the discovery of the damaging health effects caused by 'second-hand smoke' and the sense that smokers were causing 'the deaths of innocents'. The justification for stigmatising smoking is, at least in part, due to 'choice' having been established as a cornerstone of advanced liberal societies. This context paved the way for health to be popularly framed and accepted as the outcome of individual lifestyle choices and the positioning of conformity to a 'healthy lifestyle' as the logical and moral thing to do (Crawford, 1980). For example, stigma is regularly employed and felt acutely in cases where it is assumed things 'could have been otherwise': someone could have eaten healthier, avoided drug use, not harmed themselves. This is why the relative nature of choice has become central to (particularly sociological) critiques of stigmatisation. These critiques helpfully highlight how the relevance of the structural conditions under which agency, choice, and autonomy are enacted, are commonly undermined or neglected by proponents of using stigma to promote health.

In critiquing the use of stigma in public health, scholars have highlighted ethical and practical grounds for being 'anti-stigma' (Hatzenbuehler et al, 2013; Carpiniello and Pinna, 2017; Brewis and Wutich, 2019). At a micro-level, stigma promotes feelings of embarrassment, shame, and self-disgust, and associated efforts to mask 'discreditable' conditions or attributes have been shown to inhibit engagement with health behaviours, help-seeking, and accessing treatment. At a macro level, stigma has been framed as a social determinant of health that drives inequalities.

However, Bayer (2008) argues against assuming such critiques are universally applicable. He identifies the need to better define stigma, warning against 'so broadening the use of the term that it loses its bite' (Bayer, 2008, 469). For example, he draws a distinction between shaming sexual behaviours that are coercive and those that merely do not conform to conventional standards of morality. Bayer also argues it is necessary to recognise distinctions between different uses of shame. He draws on Braithwaite's (1989, 166) work on drink-driving and 'theory of re-integrative shaming', which argues 'rather than be tolerant and understanding, we should be intolerant and understanding … maintaining bonds of communication, affection, and respect rather than stigma'. Bayer's broader argument rests on a view that there is no either/or solution, but rather a perpetual need to debate the ethics of stigmatisation in different public health contexts. This is not what we see within current pro-/anti-stigma lobbies. Instead, too often, simplistic binaries in logic and morality are used in attempts to win the argument rather than understand the complexity, inconsistency, and diversity of stigma and its effects. Such binary thinking rarely delivers better understanding. We must view the pro-/anti-stigma binary more critically.

Our argument is illustrated by the example of controversial 'weight-loss guru' and self-proclaimed 'Life Bitch' Steve Miller, a hypnotherapist who provides weight-loss services. He has achieved minor celebrity in the UK as presenter of television show *Fat Families* and author of multiple weight-loss/self-help books. Miller is often invited onto mainstream media platforms to counter anti-stigma arguments and/or fat acceptance. He has described his 'disgust and impatience at society being protective of fat, lazy people' (Miller, 2007, 15). Central to his weight-loss 'methods' is getting people to accept that those who he regularly refers to as 'fatties' are lazy, irresponsible, and unattractive, and advocating for the use of disgust as motivation to lose weight.

Miller uses his lived experience as justification for his approach, citing the turning point in his own weight-loss struggles as when he decided to 'get tough' with himself. His website catalogues numerous clients who have successfully lost weight using his methods. Predictably, given the pro-/anti-stigma binary, a typical response to Miller by those who disagree with him is to deny the 'effectiveness' of his approach. Anti-weight stigma advocates tend to oppose his approach by citing research that shows exercise avoidance and emotional eating are common outcomes of stigmatising people who are fat/higher weight/living with obesity (Pearl and Puhl, 2018). They will often argue that this disproves the theory that stigma motivates weight-loss. This argument falls into the trap of accepting a false binary based on the common assumption that stigma is either good/bad, generative/inhibitory, or helpful/unhelpful. Instead, we argue that it is essential for sociological analyses to recognise and explore the diverse ways in which people experience stigma to better understand and explain its complexity and varying effects. It is highly likely that Miller and some of his clients are merely a small sample of a much larger section of society who either lose weight or maintain a 'healthy' BMI (body mass index) because they are 'motivated' by weight-related stigma – fuelled by self-hatred and/or fear of becoming fat/higher weight/living with obesity.

That stigma can have intended public health outcomes (improvements in metrics for physical health, for example) does not necessarily weaken anti-stigma arguments, nor necessarily support pro-stigma arguments. However, acknowledging this can make discussions about stigma and health more nuanced and lead to better understanding of the different ways in which people experience and respond to stigma. It leads us to ask questions about the nature of health. For example, irrespective of how effective shame and blame are in promoting physical health, what are the wider consequences of this? Simplistic binaries may give us definitive 'answers' and more certainty about the directions we should take. However, they are seldom sufficient to address complex health issues, and actively inhibit knowledge of what stigma is in any given context, where it comes from, how it impacts individual and population health, and how best to respond to it. The need to move away from pro-/anti-stigma binaries is demonstrated by our next point of discussion: anti-stigma efforts in the field of mental health.

'Destigmatisation drift': the limitations of framing stigma as *the* problem

Many, and various, anti-stigma campaigns have been released in relation to mental health, where the 'stigma' associated with a diagnosed mental illness has been blamed for a range of troubling outcomes, including: poor physical health; reduced life expectancy; low rates of help-seeking; and low-/under-employment (Pilgrim and Rogers, 2005; Hatzenbuehler et al, 2013). These anti-stigma campaigns have been subject to intense analysis and criticism. Pilgrim and Rogers (2005) argue that these campaigns are affiliated with attempts by psychiatry to bolster its professional status and a medical understanding of mental illness. For them, campaigns attempting to raise awareness and demythologise mental illness to promote health-seeking and treatment frame it as a straightforward medical issue with available and effective treatment. They argue that this serves the interests of medical professionals, which are logically and politically separate from a genuine commitment to addressing the social challenge of destigmatisation. Tyler and Slater (2018) similarly note how anti-stigma campaigns serve to individualise mental health and to obscure the need to address wider social, political, cultural, and economic conditions that produce mental distress.

Where such campaigns centre psychiatry, medicine, or a biological understanding of mental illness and addiction, they can perversely fail to reduce stigma and, in some cases, increase it. Studies show how 'biogenetic' understandings of mental illness can exacerbate or entrench stigma (Bonnington and Rose, 2014). For instance, if a mental illness is understood as genetic or biological in origin, hopes of recovery or change can be inhibited. Further, Pescosolido et al (2021) highlight that, while stigma may be reducing for some conditions (for example, depression), it is increasing or unchanged with others (for example, schizophrenia). Walsh and Foster (2020) also chart a range of unintended consequences of anti-stigma campaigns, including higher levels of fear associated with conditions that are framed as biologically based.

Anti-stigma campaigns for mental health are also critiqued for not fully considering the intersections of health conditions and inequalities (such as race, gender, and class), whether people are in safe environments to 'open up' or 'reach out', and the mismatch between urging the public to 'talk' about their mental health and the challenges faced by people who struggle to access help (Chandler, 2022). Framing the problem as stigma preventing people from openly talking about mental health implies the solution is 'breaking down' this barrier so people talk more about it. While this might be helpful for some, it significantly overestimates the public's capacity to helpfully support people with serious mental health issues or resolve the social conditions that have led to them.

These campaigns commonly frame the problems faced by those experiencing mental illness as relating to individual symptoms, and 'misunderstandings' of mental illnesses, which contribute to negative public attitudes and perceptions. Psychiatry emerges as a benevolent and caring profession, the most trusted source of knowledge about the nature of mental illness. Simultaneously, the complexity of legal, social, economic, and political struggles, and the harms that those living with mental illness may face, are disregarded. This is not to suggest that this is an either/or matter. Attempting to reverse trends in stigma by changing people's perceptions of, and attitudes towards, a condition/issue and addressing the structural factors that can determine it and/or its (non-)treatment do not need to be mutually exclusive endeavours. However, there are important, and troubling, parallels in public health between anti-stigma campaigns and the ever-popular behaviour change campaigns.

The dominance in public health of 'lifestyle' modification interventions which focus on individual behaviour change have long been the focus of critique – especially in sociology (Williams and Fullagar, 2019). It is argued that the prevailing trend of this type of 'downstream' health intervention amounts to governments abdicating responsibility for acting 'upstream' on the social determinants of health. This has been conceptualised as a policy phenomenon known as 'lifestyle drift', describing a situation whereby 'governments start with a commitment to dealing with the wider social determinants of health [such as inequality, unemployment, housing], but end up instigating narrow lifestyle interventions on individual behaviours [such as diet, physical activity]' (Hunter et al, 2010, 323).

We have conceptualised the rising popularity in anti-stigma campaigns for mental health, coupled with the well-documented failure to adequately address the structural factors that can shape mental health conditions and their (non-)treatment, as 'destigmatisation drift'. Anti-stigma campaigns can be understood to have effects akin to lifestyle drift when they shift focus away from the necessity to act on the wider determinants of health and, instead, provide governments with a relatively cheap way of demonstrating a commitment to addressing public health issues. Pleas for shifts in hearts and minds to reverse trends in stigma – that is, simply encouraging people to think differently about certain health conditions and to talk openly about them – are insufficient unless accompanied by real commitments to addressing the relevant determinants of the health conditions and their (non-)treatment. Both are needed, but it is essential to be critical when anti-stigma campaigns consistently take precedence over and/or undermine attempts to address relevant social determinants of (mental) health.

For example, Holland (2017) suggests, by contributing to the framing of the 'problem' of mental illness as one of individual attitudes, anti-stigma approaches may contribute to reasons for State disinvestment in services and social welfare. Similarly, Kapadia (2023; see also Chapter 1) argues that mental health stigma is often assumed to be inherent in racially minoritised groups. This ('cultural') framing is used to explain the 'underuse' of mental health services, with anti-stigma campaigns incorrectly sold as the solution. Kapadia (2023, 10) contends that there has been little consideration of 'the structural hierarchies and systems of power (e.g., racism) within which stigma operates' and, therefore, targeted anti-stigma campaigns are the 'wrong solution to the stigma problem'.

Bringing attention to these issues highlights that anti-stigma campaigns are frequently offered in lieu of action on the current discrepancy between demand for and provision of mental health services as well as the social conditions driving distress and suffering (such as vast inequalities in living standards). Within the current political environment, anti-stigma campaigns are liable to fall short of meeting the needs of those they are intended to benefit. Rather than simply being against anti-stigma as a concept, thinking critically about who these campaigns are attempting to support, and the nature of the support on offer, helps highlight the need to dedicate more critical attention to the theory and practice of anti-stigma.

Recalibrating anti-stigma

In critiquing the pro-/anti-stigma binary, we have sought to underline how complex and fraught with tensions stigma is when it intersects with health, illness, and public health/medicine. We now draw on three cases – 'obesity', anorexia, and self-harm – to further problematise such dualistic thinking and begin to outline priorities for recalibrating anti-stigma.

'Obesity'

The fields of critical weight studies, critical obesity studies, and fat studies, as well as activism outside of academia, have demonstrated both widespread and enduring stigmatisation of people of higher body weights/larger body sizes and the need for change (Monaghan et al, 2022). People of higher body weights are often portrayed as greedy and lazy, irresponsibly and immorally choosing personal comfort and pleasure over a supposed civic duty to manage their weight to avoid placing an unnecessary and costly burden on health services (Williams and Annandale, 2020). While much has been written about how and why weight stigma is unfair, unhelpful, and harmful (Pearl et al, 2024), what anti-stigma looks like in relation to higher body weights is complex and contested. Much of the contestation revolves around whether medicalisation/pathologisation challenges or reinforces stigma.

As a way of tackling stigma, patient advocates/organisations and pharmaceutical companies tend to argue for defining 'obesity' as a disease. For them, it is medically and morally sound, a necessary step to improve the quality and availability of healthcare, and a means to shift blame away from individuals, who can be recast as 'ill' and not entirely responsible for their body weight (Rubino et al, 2020). Conversely, those aligned with fat activism, fat acceptance, and body positivity have argued against pathologising body weight on the grounds that this is inaccurate, immoral, and an ineffective anti-stigma strategy (Spratt, 2023). It is commonly argued that weight and BMI are poor proxies for physical health, focusing on them promotes a grossly simplified understanding of health/wellbeing, and pathologising 'fat' or bigger/heavier bodies is itself stigmatising (LeBesco, 2011). It is disputed that pathologisation would, in fact, dispel stereotypical beliefs about people of higher weights/bigger sizes or result in significant investment in related healthcare. As previously noted, medicalising mental health conditions has not resolved stigma, nor led to well-resourced mental health services.

An illustrative point of tension is terminology. Meadows and Daníelsdóttir (2016) outline how fat activism, fat acceptance, and body positivity movements have long advocated for using the term 'fat' – reclaiming it as a neutral descriptor to counter its widespread use as a pejorative term. As with discriminatory terms relating to race, disability, and sexuality being reclaimed by communities who they were/are used against, many argue that reclaiming 'fat' to describe oneself and others should be understood and experienced as an act of unity and empowerment. In contrast, patient advocates/organisations and pharmaceutical companies tend to frame 'fat' as offensive and have advocated using medical terminology and adopting person-first language ('person with obesity', rather than 'obese person'). The principle of person-first language originates from the disability movement in the 1990s, where people campaigned not to be defined by their disability. Person-first language is now mandatory in many spaces in the obesity field and seen as an important part of adopting an anti-stigma/ non-stigmatising approach. These approaches to addressing stigma are clearly irreconcilable. Despite both seeking to counteract stigma, universal application of either terminology would be experienced as stigmatising for some. Meadows and Daníelsdóttir (2016, 1) recognise this irreconcilability, arguing that 'it is unlikely there can ever be agreement between people whose "solution" to body diversity is social justice and acceptance of this diversity, and those whose "solution" is elimination of the difference [via weight-loss/-management]'. The playing out of these tensions highlights how anti-stigma campaigning is not as it is often portrayed – that is, those who are anti-stigma taking on those who are consciously pro-stigma and/or educating those who unconsciously stigmatise.

These debates demonstrate the challenges of more simplistic readings of 'anti-stigma' campaigning, showing how different groups of stigmatised people can end up competing to define what is and is not stigmatising, and how best to respond to this. As such, anti-stigma campaigns can ultimately privilege the needs and preferences of some over others and, potentially, reproduce or exacerbate inequalities and entrench discrimination against already marginalised groups. For example, Bombak (2023) demonstrates how pharmaceutical companies, as part of a pro-pathologisation approach to higher weights, have directed considerable attention and resources to establishing themselves as authorities on weight stigma. Against the backdrop of the development, approval, and widespread distribution of weight-loss drugs, Bombak documents how pharmaceutical companies have co-opted and distorted fat activism to define weight stigma along lines that serve their interests instead (pathologising higher weights). Bombak (2023, 858) contends that 'a discourse has now emerged in which opposition to the pharmaceuticalization of "obesity" is labelled stigmatizing'. She warns that, because there are contrasting views on whether higher weights should be pathologised, 'it is essential that powerful and well-moneyed corporations are not in control of how we come to understand the bodily diversity that surrounds us' (Bombak, 2023, 860).

Anorexia and 'pro-ana'

People with eating disorders regularly experience harmful stereotypes, prejudice, and discrimination. Research on 'eating disorder stigma' demonstrates a common public perception (also evident in healthcare) that eating disorders are self-inflicted and result from people acting irresponsibly. Brelet et al's (2021) review of this research indicates that stigma can exacerbate eating disorders and delay recovery. Clearly there is a need to counter stigma in this area. However, the 'pro-ana' community – an online grassroots response to stigma associated with anorexia – is a controversial example that highlights the complexity and moral ambiguity of addressing this stigma.

It is difficult to define the 'pro-ana' community as there is not a 'universally coherent standpoint' across it (Yeshua-Katz, 2015, 1348). Broadly speaking, pro-ana can be understood as a response to, and resistance of, the stigmatisation of anorexia. Community members often claim that being pro-ana counteracts being misunderstood, being mischaracterised, and/or lacking support. Yet, how members choose to counteract this differs wildly. For some, it involves rejecting the biomedical model, emphasising choice, and positively reframing who they are and how they live. For others, it is asserting that anorexia is a medical condition, educating others that it is not simply something someone irresponsibly chooses to do, and seeking support from others who struggle/struggled with it.

Yeshua-Katz and Martins' (2013) research on those who embrace the medicalisation of their condition and seek non-judgemental support highlights a 'pro-ana paradox', whereby blogging about anorexia both alleviated and triggered anxiety. Blogging was cathartic and opened up social support, but also prompted fears about exacerbating their condition, encouraging disordered eating in others, and impeding recovery for themselves and others. However, it was those who rejected the biomedical model and, to some extent, celebrated and promoted a 'pro-ana lifestyle' who were subject to most controversy, and prompted calls to censor pro-ana blogs. This has led to the pro-ana community being referred to as 'doubly stigmatised': facing stigma associated with anorexia *and* considered to be stigmatised as a perceived threat to the health of others (Yeshua-Katz, 2015).

In 2012, several popular blog-hosting services announced they would censor content perceived to promote self-harm (including eating disorders). This decision followed significant pressure from eating disorder organisations, people with lived experience of eating disorders, and families who were bereaved or supporting family members with eating disorders (Schott et al, 2016). The potential for pro-ana spaces to be inclusive, educational, and supportive responses to stigma became overshadowed by content: offering and asking for 'thinspiration'/'thinspo' (pictures of emaciated people to inspire commitment to weight-loss efforts); 'tips and tricks' for losing weight/maintaining low weights, disguising what others labelled dangerous behaviour, and resisting medical intervention/recovery; and group activities to facilitate/motivate the achievement of an authentic anorexic look/identity (Norris et al, 2006; Boero and Pascoe, 2012).

Demonstrating authenticity was central to pro-ana communities and crucial for another key feature: policing membership. Policing was not primarily to provide 'safe spaces' that protect members from outsiders enacting stigma/abuse, as is more usual in anti-stigma work. This policing, instead, served to aggressively establish who the 'real' or 'true' 'pro-ana anorexics' were and who could be excluded and denigrated on the basis of being a 'wannarexic' (Boero and Pascoe, 2012). As Boero and Pascoe (2012, 39) explain, accusations of 'wannarexic' are a common feature of pro-ana communities; it is the 'ultimate insult, as it implies a person does not belong' and is not sufficiently anorexic. Such accusations can be seen to set entry standards for others to aspire to and emulate. It is in keeping with common experiences of anorexia as hierarchical and competitive. This has been documented to transform inpatient settings into places where patients compete to be the most ill and paradoxically learn how to 'get better at' rather than 'better from' anorexia (Warin, 2010; O'Connell, 2023). So, unlike other anti-stigma practices, a central feature of many pro-ana communities in these studies was shaming others. If stigma involves labelling others as less valuable, undesirable, or unwanted (Brewis and Wutich, 2019), the aggressive outing and ridiculing of 'wannarexics' can be seen as the *stigmatised* turned *stigmatisers*. Nonetheless, the pro-ana community might argue instead that this is a vehicle for members to resist and reverse stigma – that is, not by attempting to stop others from stigmatising anorexia, but by ascribing value to, and actively encouraging, it.

Calls to censor pro-ana sites on these grounds are understandable. However, they are not without controversy or consequence. Schott et al (2016, 108, 110) argue that censoring pro-ana sites is 'muzzling expression', because 'they represent meaningful opportunities for women and girls to share their experiences, confront the issues that they face, and find ways to support one another'. In addition, Cobb's (2017) analysis demonstrates that an unintended consequence of censorship has been the integration of pro-ana content into the mainstream. Taking examples such as the use of #thinspo and #bonespo on social media after the ban, Cobb (2017, 199) illustrates how pro-ana users can hide in plain sight by 'disguising their spaces as weight loss motivation blogs and drawing on discourses of health to legitimise them'. Cobb (2017, 201) ultimately contends that the normalisation of pro-ana content demonstrates 'the extent to which what constitutes healthy body practices in the mainstream is often indistinguishable from that which has been framed as disordered'.

It is clearly limited to present pro-ana content as 'the problem' when prevailing societal trends actively promote the aesthetic of thinness that drives many eating disorders. Though, it is possible to be critical of both social drivers of eating disorders *and* online practices that actively encourage, facilitate, and entrench anorexia. Pro-ana is not discussed here to argue what a suitable anti-stigma response to anorexia stigma should be. Rather, this example highlights the often under-acknowledged complexity of anti-stigma practice. What it means to be 'anti-stigma', in relation to anorexia, is unclear. Can someone be anti-stigma if they are not pro-ana? Can anti-stigma practice encompass exclusionary and abusive spaces that actively promote and facilitate harm? More generally, anti-stigma practice is focused on harm reduction/eradication. Pro-ana challenges this and highlights that what it means to be anti-stigma in relation to self-harm requires more critical attention.

Self-harm

Self-harm is a practice understood as related to mental illness and is characterised as inherently 'stigmatised' (Long, 2018). The stigmatised nature of self-harm is reflected in those who self-harm experiencing social exclusion and poor or abusive treatment in medical settings, and the practice often being kept hidden with help-seeking avoided (McShane, 2012; Chandler, 2016, 2018). This has been met with routine attempts to 'tackle' self-harm stigma, often as part of 'anti-stigma' campaigns for mental health focused on educating the public. For instance, a study by suicide prevention charity Samaritans (2023) examined perceptions of self-harm among different groups with and without experience of self-harm. They identified widespread stigma, including over half of their respondents stating they would not 'carpool' or rent an apartment to someone who had self-harmed. The report recommendations focused on educating the public about self-harm and the impact of stigma. This approach is typical and exemplifies the 'destigmatisation drift' identified earlier in the chapter. It does little to address the structural conditions that may shape self-harm stigma (and exacerbate its impact for some groups more than others), nor does it engage with *why* self-harm attracts such negative perceptions and responses. Seemingly the assumption is that, if only people understood both self-harm and the negative impacts of stigma better, their behaviour/attitudes and, relatedly, the lives of those who self-harm, would improve. This is questionable.

Anti-stigma approaches to self-harm are not straightforward. *Understanding* self-harm looks different for different people. This is clear in the following two examples: 1) the ongoing controversy surrounding communication about self-harm online; and 2) the management of self-harm in therapeutic relationships and settings.

Tensions surrounding self-harm content online were starkly illustrated in 2018 when Instagram began to moderate self-harm-related posts, in response to concerns that viewing such content caused harm to 'vulnerable people' (particularly young women). The moderation extended to removing images showing self-harm scars as well as more confronting images of wounds/cuts. Stirling and Chandler (2020) write about the discomfort of realising that their scarred arms were deemed 'dangerous' to others. Similarly, academics, activists, and practitioners reflected in a blog series on the complex issues this 'ban' provoked (The Sociological Review, 2019). Critics of the 'ban' argued that people who self-harmed often benefitted from communicating openly about self-harm online, including sharing images – especially of healed/

healing scars. Concerns were raised about the 'ban' exacerbating stigma, deeming self-harmed bodies as clearly taboo, to be hidden and ashamed of. In contrast, fears were raised about the potential for such images and communication to encourage self-harm in others and normalise it. This reflected a shift from framing self-harm not only as a stigmatised practice, but towards viewing the self-harmed body (and by extension, the self-harming person) as themselves a 'risk to others' as well as themselves. By showing images online, and normalising self-harm, they may inadvertently encourage 'vulnerable' persons to engage in the practice. Charities and researchers often call for a balanced approach that recognises the potential for online content to be helpful or harmful for different people (Lavis and Winter, 2020; Marsh et al, 2022).

Tensions have continued to intensify, with debates relating to the UK Online Harms Act (2023), and media coverage of the death of Molly Russell, widely attributed to self-harm content on Instagram. These raise crucial questions about the relationship between normalisation and anti-stigma initiatives, and whether it is possible to be 'anti-stigma' without also normalising a given practice. Certainly, mainstream approaches to anti-stigma suggest this is possible, arguing both that self-harm is stigmatised and requires greater 'understanding' *and* that communication about self-harm (especially online) needs to be undertaken with care to avoid 'normalising' or 'triggering' self-harm in others. How this is achieved in practice is neither clear nor straightforward.

These tensions also surface in the management of self-harm in treatment, especially inpatient hospital settings. In the 1990s/2000s, amidst much debate, there was cautious advocacy for approaches that 'allowed' self-harm (primarily via self-cutting), and in some cases 'safer self-harm' kits were provided in inpatient settings (Gutridge, 2010). These resonated strongly with user- and survivor-led approaches, which had long argued that 'stopping' self-harm may not be possible or desirable for many, and that to develop supportive or therapeutic relationships, self-harm should be seen as necessary or acceptable in some cases (Inckle, 2017). By reframing self-harm as a practice that may be helpful, and might be undertaken relatively 'safely', there is an attempt to challenge self-harm stigma. We see, here, a particular understanding of self-harm (as a '(sometimes) legitimate coping method') being advocated both to support 'treatment' and to challenge 'stigma'. However, such a move can also be seen to advocate the normalisation of self-harm – at least for some people, in some places.

What might an 'anti-stigma' approach to self-harm look like if it did not also include some aspect of 'normalisation'? This remains a hugely contested area, with stark disagreements among people with lived/living experiences of self-harm, clinical professionals, researchers, and policy makers. Understanding what self-harm means to these different (and overlapping) groups is crucial, as is closer engagement with the political economy of self-harm stigma. Absent in existing discussions is a clearer engagement with the roles of gender, race, age, and class in shaping meanings of self-harm, including the stigma associated with it. The fears that are articulated relating to normalisation, for instance, appear to centre the self-harming practices of young, White, middle-class women. We urgently need a more deeply sociological approach to self-harm stigma (and 'anti-stigma'), one that takes seriously both the micro-level aspects of how stigma is enacted in relation to self-harm (Long, 2018) and the structural factors that shape this (Chandler, 2022).

Conclusion

Through these cases, and the chapter as a whole, we have attempted to highlight three interrelated issues. First, what is considered and experienced as stigma/stigmatising is contested, not fixed. 'Anti-stigma' is often positioned as better (both morally and practically) than alternatives, yet too little critical attention has been dedicated to who determines how stigma is defined and should be countered, and who benefits from (or is disadvantaged by) a particular understanding and framing of (anti-)stigma in any given context. Second, people resist and oppose stigma in different ways, and this diversity of resistance/opposition will not always be morally coherent or consistent in effect. While anti-stigma and 'pro-condition' positions will overlap, more critical attention is required to explore where the overlaps are, and in what instances they diverge. Third, anti-stigma efforts are designed to promote destigmatisation, but reducing harm at an individual level may increase harm at a population level. Can this be mitigated? Does destigmatisation lead inevitably to normalisation and what are the consequences either way? These are important questions that need to be engaged with critically.

None of these inquiries are well-served by a pro-/anti-stigma binary and accompanying lobbies. These binary positions betray the complexity, inconsistency, and diversity of stigma and its effects in and on public health. Although moral certainty can be appealing – and there are certainly moral grounds for objecting to the personal suffering/harm and creation/perpetuation of social inequalities and injustices caused by stigma – this is not enough to justify limiting our understanding of what stigma is and does through oversimplification. Our aim has been to demonstrate why anti-stigma work in mental health should act as a warning. What we have conceptualised as destigmatisation drift is already happening and is likely to become more widespread. While there are powerful forces at play in the restricted remit of public health, the pro-/anti-stigma binary has informed the underdevelopment of anti-stigma theory and practice, and this is damaging efforts to address social drivers of stigma, illness, distress, and suffering.

As sociologists researching stigma, we are committed to challenging and addressing stigma to reduce suffering and promote health and wellbeing. We see this critique of anti-stigma as serving these ends. Despite what those who endorse the pro-/anti-stigma binary may advocate, understanding and addressing stigma is far from straightforward morally or practically. It is crucial, then, that the recalibration of stigma includes a recalibration of anti-stigma.

Could things be different?

- Not thinking in terms of being pro- or anti-stigma could help move people away from oversimplistic ideas about what stigma is, what it does, and how its potential to cause harm can be limited.
- There must be greater recognition that in any given context a 'one-size-fits-all' approach to anti-stigma is likely to be inappropriate and inadequate. Attempts to engage with groups considered to be stigmatised could instead work with the reality that stigma is not understood or experienced by everyone in the same way.
- Highlighting that anti-stigma campaigns are not inherently positive could build public support for more meaningful social change. This would help people to expect more from anti-stigma campaigns – by promoting opposition to public health agencies (and others) conveniently framing stigma as 'the problem' and by creating opportunities to call for more significant action on the social factors that drive illness, suffering, and stigma.

References

Bayer, R. (2008) 'Stigma and the ethics of public health: Not can we but should we', *Social Science and Medicine*, 67(3): 463–72.

Boero, N. and Pascoe, C.J. (2012) 'Pro-anorexia communities and online interaction: Bringing the pro-ana body online', *Body and Society*, 18(2): 27–57.

Bombak, A. (2023) 'How pharmaceutical companies misappropriate fat acceptance', *Critical Public Health*, 33(5): 856–63.

Bonnington, O. and Rose, D. (2014) 'Exploring stigmatisation among people diagnosed with either bipolar disorder or borderline personality disorder: A critical realist analysis', *Social Science and Medicine*, 123(0): 7–17.

Braithwaite, J. (1989) *Crime, Shame and Reintegration*, Cambridge: Cambridge University Press.

Brelet, L., Flaudias, V., Désert, M., Guillaume, S., Llorca, P.M. and Boirie, Y. (2021) 'Stigmatization toward people with anorexia nervosa, bulimia nervosa, and binge eating disorder: A scoping review', *Nutrients*, 13(8): 2834.

Brewis, A. and Wutich, A. (2019) *Lazy, Crazy, and Disgusting: Stigma and the Undoing of Global Health*, Baltimore: Johns Hopkins University Press.

Carpiniello, B. and Pinna, F. (2017) 'The reciprocal relationship between suicidality and stigma', *Frontiers in Psychiatry*, 8: 35.

Chandler, A. (2016) *Self-Injury, Medicine and Society: Authentic Bodies*, Basingstoke: Palgrave Macmillan.

Chandler, A. (2018) 'Seeking secrecy: A qualitative study of younger adolescents' accounts of self-harm', *YOUNG: Nordic Journal of Youth Research*, 26(4): 313–31.

Chandler, A. (2022) 'Masculinities and suicide: Unsettling "talk" as a response to suicide in men', *Critical Public Health*, 32(4): 499–508.

Cobb, G. (2017) '"This is not pro-ana": Denial and disguise in pro-anorexia online spaces', *Fat Studies*, 6(2): 189–205.

Crawford, R. (1980) 'Healthism and the medicalization of everyday life', *International Journal of Health Services*, 10(3): 365–88.

Goffman, E. (1963) *Stigma: Notes on the Management of Spoiled Identity*, New York: Penguin.

Gutridge, K. (2010) 'Safer self-injury or assisted self-harm?', *Theoretical Medicine and Bioethics*, 31(1): 79–92.

Hatzenbuehler, M.L., Phelan, J.C. and Link, B.G. (2013) 'Stigma as a fundamental cause of population health inequalities', *American Journal of Public Health*, 103(5): 813–21.

Holland, K. (2017) 'Biocommunicability and the politics of mental health: An analysis of responses to the ABC's "Mental As" campaign', *Communication Research and Practice*, 3(2): 176–93.

Hunter, D.J., Popay, J., Tannahill, C. and Whitehead, M. (2010) 'Getting to grips with health inequalities at last?: Marmot review calls for renewed action to create a fairer society', *BMJ*, 340: 323–4.

Inckle, K. (2017) *Safe with Self-Injury: A Practical Guide to Understanding, Responding and Harm-Reduction*, Monmouth: PCCS Books.

Kapadia, D. (2023) 'Stigma, mental illness and ethnicity: Time to centre racism and structural stigma', *Sociology of Health and Illness*, 45(4): 855–71.

Lavis, A. and Winter, R. (2020) '#Online harms or benefits? An ethnographic analysis of the positives and negatives of peer-support around self-harm on social media', *Journal of Child Psychology and Psychiatry*, 61(8): 842–54.

LeBesco, K. (2011) 'Neoliberalism, public health, and the moral perils of fatness', *Critical Public Health*, 21(2): 153–64.

Long, M. (2018) '"We're not monsters … we're just really sad sometimes:" Hidden self-injury, stigma and help-seeking', *Health Sociology Review*, 27(1): 89–103.

Marsh, I., Winter, R. and Marzano, L. (2022) 'Representing suicide: Giving voice to a desire to die?', *Health*, 26(1): 10–26.

McShane, T. (2012) *Blades, Blood and Bandages: The Experiences of People who Self-Injure*, Basingstoke: Palgrave Macmillan.

Meadows, A. and Daníelsdóttir, S. (2016) 'What's in a word? On weight stigma and terminology', *Frontiers in Psychology*, 7: 1527.

Miller, S. (2007) *Get Off Your Arse and Lose Weight: Straight-Talking Advice on How to Get Thin from the Life Bitch!*, London: Headline Publishing Group.

Monaghan, L.F., Rich, E. and Bombak, A.E. (2022) *Rethinking Obesity: Critical Perspectives in Crisis Times*, Abingdon: Routledge.

Norris, M.L., Boydell, K.M., Pinhas, L. and Katzman, D.K. (2006) 'Ana and the internet: A review of pro-anorexia websites', *International Journal of Eating Disorders*, 39(6): 443–7.

O'Connell, L. (2023) 'Being and doing anorexia nervosa: An autoethnography of diagnostic identity and performance of illness', *Health*, 27(2): 263–78.

Pearl, R.L. and Puhl, R.M. (2018) 'Weight bias internalization and health: A systematic review', *Obesity Reviews*, 19(8): 1141–63.

Pearl, R.L., Donze, L.F., Rosas, L.G., Agurs-Collins, T., Baskin, M.L., Breland, J.Y. et al (2024) 'Ending weight stigma to advance health equity', *American Journal of Preventive Medicine*, 67(5): 785–91.

Pescosolido, B.A., Halpern-Manners, A., Luo, L. and Perry, B. (2021) 'Trends in public stigma of mental illness in the US, 1996–2018', *JAMA Network Open*, 4(12): e2140202.

Pilgrim, D. and Rogers, A.E. (2005) 'Psychiatrists as social engineers: A study of an anti-stigma campaign', *Social Science and Medicine*, 61(12): 2546–56.

Rubino, F., Puhl, R.M., Cummings, D.E., Eckel, R.H., Ryan, D.H., Mechanick, J.I. et al (2020) 'Joint international consensus statement for ending stigma of obesity', *Nature Medicine*, 26(4): 485–97.

Samaritans (2023) *An Open Secret: Self-Harm and Stigma in Ireland and Northern Ireland*, Dublin: Samaritans Ireland.

Scambler, G. (2018) 'Heaping blame on shame: "Weaponising stigma" for neoliberal times', *The Sociological Review*, 66(4): 766–82.

Schott, N.D., Spring, L. and Langan, D. (2016) 'Neoliberalism, pro-ana/mia websites, and pathologizing women: Using performance ethnography to challenge psychocentrism', *Studies in Social Justice*, 10(1): 95–115.

Spratt, T. (2023) 'Understanding "fat shaming" in a neoliberal era: Performativity, healthism and the UK's "obesity epidemic"', *Feminist Theory*, 24(1): 86–101.

Stirling, F.J. and Chandler, A. (2020) 'Dangerous arms and everyday activism: A dialogue between two researchers with lived experience of self-harm', *International Review of Qualitative Research*, 14(1): 155–70.

The Sociological Review (2019) 'Self-harm', *The Sociological Review*, [online], Available from: https://thesociologicalreview.org/collections/self-harm/ [Accessed 30 January 2025].

Tyler, I. and Slater, T. (2018). 'Rethinking the sociology of stigma', *The Sociological Review*, 66(4): 721–43.

Walsh, D.A.B. and Foster, J.L.H. (2020) 'A call to action: A critical review of mental health related anti-stigma campaigns', *Frontiers in Public Health*, 8: 569539.

Warin, M. (2010) *Abject Relations: Everyday Worlds of Anorexia*, New Brunswick: Rutgers University Press.

Williams, O. and Annandale, E. (2020) 'Obesity, stigma and reflexive embodiment: Feeling the "weight" of expectation', *Health*, 24(4): 421–41.

Williams, O. and Fullagar, S. (2019) 'Lifestyle drift and the phenomenon of "citizen shift" in contemporary UK health policy', *Sociology of Health and Illness*, 41(1): 20–35.

Yeshua-Katz, D. (2015) 'Online stigma resistance in the pro-ana community', *Qualitative Health Research*, 25(10): 1347–58.

Yeshua-Katz, D. and Martins, N. (2013) 'Communicating stigma: The pro-ana paradox', *Health Communication*, 28(5): 499–508.

7

Readdressing Addiction Stigma: Making Space for Being in the World Differently

Fay Dennis

Introduction

> There was no problem with the drugs. Heroin has done no harm to me. Everything else has, like the lifestyle and whatever has, but not the actual drug. (James [pseudonym], a research participant, heroin user and harm reductionist, 2019)

> By shifting our relations to the characteristics we are being made to see as [the disease problem], we can refigure them as ways of being in the world differently, and as such, as other ways of being human. (Latimer, 2018, 848)

In shifting 'the problem' of drugs from the drug or person who uses them to the environment in which they are consumed, James speaks to an argument made by Joanna Latimer (2018) in her discussion of dementia stigma. Latimer argues that by shifting our relations to the characteristics we see as the disease problem, in her case, dementia, but here, the problem of dependent drug use or addiction, we can refigure them as ways of *being in the world* differently. What is appealing about this approach is its hopefulness for a world where people who use drugs dependently can be more accepted and able to pursue and inhabit identities more easily alongside 'drug user' or 'addict'. This is not to say that frequent, heavy drug use is not a problem for many people. But, by relocating where 'the problem' comes from, we make space for those like James and many in the harm reduction movement who do not automatically see it in these terms. And, if listened to, they may be able to shed light on alternative, less stigmatising relationships with drugs. For its potential to disrupt disease categories, this argument goes further than mainstream anti-addiction stigma work.

Through the stories of people who use drugs (predominantly heroin and/or crack cocaine) in my research in London, UK, I have come to think about stigma, that is, the 'discrediting' (Goffman, 1963) problem of drug consumption, relationally in terms of how people who use drugs are blocked in their ability to be in the world (quite literally to be alive and well, and to be able to pursue different activities and roles). Like Goffman (1963) argued in his classic sociological work, stigma is not inherent to the person but rather produced and sustained through social relations. I look at how this stigma takes place through three stories of what I call, following Deleuzo-Guattarian (1987) thinking, 'blocked becoming'. These stories account for how people are constrained by their 'association' with drugs and addiction and the narrow understanding of the human that addiction is rooted in (based on autonomy and volition). It is, therefore, not the drug–body interaction but these more complicated socio-material relationships that prevent people who use drugs from living full lives.

If we see being with drugs as different ways of being human, we can ask what more we can do to enable flourishing rather than what more we can do to make people give up. This is what is at the very heart of the harm reduction movement and ethos – an acceptance of different ways of being. This approach is in sharp contrast with the predominance of abstinence-based recovery programmes, where elimination of drug use is considered the only legitimate/successful way to 'treat' drug addiction/dependency. And this is what James' realisation is about. He explains how he spent ten years trying to get off drugs – on a cycle of abstinence and relapse – until, one day, 'the penny dropped':

> Becoming abstinent, getting a job, relapsing … I went around and around on this wheel for about 10 years until, probably four or five years ago, the penny dropped. I don't know why, but it was, 'I'm not doing any harm to anybody. I'm not a thief, what's the problem?' It was like a weight lifted off my chest.

In questioning and dislocating 'the problem' – one that he was told to see in the drugs, in his dependency, and ultimately in himself – a huge weight was lifted: 'It was other people's feelings put onto me and I kind of believed that shit. When I just sat down and actually looked at it, 'What harm am I doing?' When I realised that, it all just went away.' Suddenly, he no longer had to live a life of shame trying to get off drugs and failing. His involvement with harm reduction activism provided him with this acceptance: 'Most of that came about through getting involved in the activism side of things. That's just really opened my eyes up to so much. I have no issues at all to do with drug use at all now, at all.' James no longer viewed himself as a failed person, but somebody living a different kind of life to one normatively judged as acceptable. The harm and problem he once saw as coming from the drug and himself he now locates within these judging others, and his positioning as an outsider where his practices are outlawed and pushed underground, exposing him to an unregulated drug market, criminal violence, and overdose risk. James now takes a different approach to his drug use, seeing methadone, an opioid used in heroin treatment, as any other medication (that is, to aid living as somebody who uses drugs rather than to 'recover' a former non-addicted self), and heroin as 'a glass of brandy … at the end of the night':

> I don't particularly have any treatment aims. I see the methadone now basically as I take tablets for my stomach, dyspepsia or something. It's just another medication. I don't think I must stop, or I must get off methadone.

> [Heroin is] like a glass of brandy, somebody having a cigar at the end of the night or whatever.

In shifting the relations to what we normally see as addiction — to the substance, and to the daily need for it — James enters a more harmonious relationship with his drug use and treatment. The daily need for methadone is reframed as like anyone else's need for daily medication, and the desire for heroin is likened to how other people might desire recreational, legal drugs for relaxation. This likening to mainstream, majoritarian societal interests and actors actively resists a positioning of the addict as Other. He explains how he no longer has these 'hang-ups' about being a 'heroin user and a drug addict'. This is because, in many ways, he is no longer (if he ever was) 'an addict' as it has been taught to him — uncontrolled, compulsive, a thief, and harmful to others. In shifting this perspective, he has freed how he sees himself from this stigmatising identity and, crucially, the suffering, anguish, and guilt that has come with it.

In this chapter, I want to further tease out some of the ways that the category of addiction works to block what people can become and explore openings for alternative configurations with drugs. Therefore, this is not simply about the stigma associated with addiction, but the stigmatising which may be inherent to addiction as a disease category. In this sense, the argument is different to anti-stigma work which attempts to disentangle stigma from addiction, and, indeed, even looks to addiction to destigmatise people who use drugs, thereby replacing a moral category with a pathological one. Instead, following Deleuze and Guattari (1987), and as made relevant to the drugs field by Peta Malins (2004), I observe the socio-material ways that body-persons are stratified as addicts – discussed in what follows as 'junkie', 'thief', and 'prostitute' – and their 'blocking' effect. As James explains, it is not the drug or dependency that has meant he has to live a stigmatised life on 'this wheel' of abstinence and relapse, but these associations and 'other people's feelings put onto [him]'. Rather than judging from the outside, then, I want to ask what can be learned from this insider perspective – turning the gaze inward to ask, where is the stigmatising problem of addiction coming from?

Addiction stigma

Stigma is regularly discussed in the literature on addiction and dependent drug use. These works can be seen to fall into two groups. The first group tends to separate stigma from the category of addiction, which is either left unchecked or endorsed as a mode of destigmatising people who use drugs. The second group takes a more critical approach both to the social and political roots of addiction stigma, and to the category of addiction itself, which is seen to go to the very heart of the stigma facing people who use drugs.

Addressing the first group, scholars have focused on the specificities and experience of stigma rather than its origins as a social process. These studies largely draw on theories of phenomenology and social psychology in exploring the lived experience of addiction stigma (Radcliffe and Stevens, 2008; Simmonds and Coomber, 2009; Kulesza et al, 2013). Scholars have also actively endorsed and engaged with the concept of addiction as a way out of stigma. This follows the disease model of addiction and the idea that seeing heavy, dependent drug use as a brain disease removes blame from the individual and supports a health-based approach. Within this guise, stigma is seen as a by-product of a moral ideology on drugs as *bad* and their users as personally flawed and lacking self-control. Thus, education around addiction as a disease is judged to be what is needed to tackle stigma and improve the lives of people who use drugs. A leading proponent of the disease model of addiction, Nora Volkow (director of the National Institute of Drug Abuse in the United States, the largest funder of drug research globally), explained in 2015:

> If we embrace the concept of addiction as a chronic disease where drugs have disrupted the most fundamental circuits that enable us to do something that we take for granted – make a decision and follow it through – we will be able to decrease the stigma, not just in the lay public, but in the health care system, among providers and insurers. (Fraser et al, 2017, 193)

Such thinking can be seen to inform recent public health campaigns in the UK like the National Health Service (NHS) Addiction Provider Alliance's (2022) campaign, 'Stigma Kills', which aims to 'break down the myths and misconceptions around addiction demonstrating it is both a mental and physical health condition and not a person's choice'. But, following Suzanne Fraser and colleagues, as sociologists of health and illness, it is hard to believe that disease labelling can lead to less stigma. As these authors note, '[i]t is becoming evident that labelling addiction a brain disease and then attempting to "educate" the public about this disease is not producing any consistent change in stigmatising perspectives' (Fraser et al, 2017, 194). Considering the proliferation of stigma that still exists as depicted in the lived experience of people who use drugs, this emphasis does not seem to be making the promised difference. Indeed, for historian of addiction Nancy Campbell (2023) the brain disease model is simply a reinvention of the moral model.

The second group of literature is informed by a more critical take on the category of addiction and the social and political roots of addiction stigma. One way of thinking about the politics and power of addiction stigma that has particularly risen to significance in recent years is through a re/turn to a Marxist lens of political economy and structure, what Imogen Tyler (2018, 2020) calls 'the stigma machine'. This style of thinking is taken up in Addison et al's (2022) edited book, *Drugs, Identity and Stigma*. Quoting Tyler (2018), they argue that stigma constitutes a cacophony of 'mechanisms of inequality' as a 'site of social and political struggle over value' which enables profiteering and deters people from making claims on the State (Addison et al, 2022, 2–3). Such an interest is also taken forward in Liviu Alexandrescu's (forthcoming) book, *Drugscapes: Imaginaries of Intoxication, Dependency, and Control*, in which he explores the ways addiction is 'mobilised in the moral imaginary by the powerful against the powerless to justify the unjust orders of a deeply unequal social world'. In this mode of inquiry, researchers are asked to 'gaze up' (Paton, 2018), including to the very work of the campaigns that seek to challenge stigma (Tyler and Slater, 2018, 727). For example, Alexandrescu (forthcoming) explores the role of pharmaceutical companies in stigmatising pain, which is seen to be at the heart of the US opioid crisis.

Where we have seen scholars 'gaze up' to the stigmatisers – those structures and organisations producing and standing to gain from stigma – and others down to the stigmatised in accounts of lived experience, there are yet some who argue for a third way based on:

> The mutual co-production of power and subjectivity, placing stigma into a performative ontological framework more attentive to the socially constitutive role of such phenomena and, we think, allowing useful insights into stigma's ubiquity and persistence. (Fraser et al, 2017, 194)

Turning the gaze inwards, then, addiction plays an important role in contemporary liberal societies precisely as a mode of Othering. In this register, addiction 'is a means by which contemporary liberal subjects are schooled and disciplined in the forms of conduct and dispositions required to belong, and to count as fully human' (Fraser et al, 2017, 199). For Jarret Zigon (2019, 53), ' "the addict" has been rendered as the dangerous internal Other from whom the population must be defended'. Addicts are 'those who have lost the characteristics that today are equated with humanness: their freedom, autonomy, self-responsibility, and control' (Zigon, 2019, 60). Taking up this third way, then, I continue to gaze inwards, asking where stigma is coming from and how best to apprehend it.

My approach

The stigma of addiction is a truism that is often left unexplained in the literature on drugs. In their recent review of stigma and hepatitis C, an infectious disease associated with injecting drug use, Harris et al (2021, 2) note: 'While commonly employed as a framing concept, much research lacks explicit theoretical or critical engagement on how stigma is conceptualised'. Moreover, stigma has become somewhat of a catch-all term for the disadvantage and discrimination experienced by people who use drugs, especially in terms of accessing services. It also becomes a convenient way of distracting attention away from underfunding and under-resourcing, what Graham Scambler (2018) refers to as the 'weaponising of stigma' in neoliberal times. For example, in a recent radio interview (BBC Radio 4, 2022) with a government minister for Scotland on the growing use and deaths associated with illicit benzodiazepine, we are relayed a deeply disturbing story from a mother whose son nearly died while suffering psychosis linked to his benzodiazepine use. He was put into an induced coma, only to be discharged from hospital two days later because there were no beds at a neighbouring psychiatric unit. In a sudden and frankly insensitive response to this desperate situation, the minister brings up stigma. Nowhere in this mother's story was there mention of stigma. Her son was not refused help because of stigma. He was refused help because there was no space for him. In this jarring moment, we see how the language and concept of stigma can be employed (even if unknowingly) to cover over and divert attention away from structural inequality and government inaction.

For these reasons, I have tended to avoid the term stigma in my work, especially where it appears relatively stable (as a weapon to be drawn on) and outside of socioeconomic processes. Here, then, I engage with the specificities of where drug events become stigmatising or produce stigmatising effects, and think of stigma as always relational and in process. Speaking to this relationship in her extensive work on Deleuzo-Guattarian approaches, Peta Malins (2004, 88) explains how drug-using bodies become blocked and identities become fixed:

Most often a drug using body is connected … to the social machines of public health or medicine or morality through which it becomes stratified as a 'drug user' or 'addict' or 'deviant' respectively. Or the machine of law, through which it becomes stratified as a 'criminal' (or now, through diversionary programs: a 'recovering addict'!). Or it might, if we allow it, connect up to a multitude of other machines and become something else entirely (a student, an architect, a mother, a surfer, a masochist, a gardener, a knitter).

In this chapter, I focus on three striking accounts of where participants discuss their stratifications as a 'junkie', 'thief', and 'prostitute', and the ways that they are blocked, respectively, from becoming a patient, a guest at a party, and an employee. As will become clear, it is in these stratifying connections – of imagery, legislation, knowledge, and objects – that body-persons are blocked (from becoming *other than* an addict). Thought of in this way, stigma is a relational activity that keeps people trapped in the addict identity, plugged into these webs of control.

This is different from Goffman's relational approach, in which he focuses too much on the affected individuals and how they cope and relate to others, and not enough on 'why particular features or issues come to be stigmatised' and what is achieved politically by this stigmatisation (Fraser et al, 2017, 194), or the 'bigger picture', as Tyler (2018, 2020) puts it (see also Parker and Aggleton, 2003; Hannem and Brucket, 2012; Addison et al, 2022). But so too is the approach taken here different from a solely top-down approach of the powerful over the powerless where people who use drugs can easily be rendered passive. What draws me, then, to understanding stigma through Deleuze and Guattari's ontology of becoming is its inherent hopefulness, to 'become something else' (and hold multiple identities), as Malins (2004) phrases it.

Blocked becomings: stratified as a 'junkie', 'thief', and 'prostitute'

Beckie (B): [My partner] died on my lap … He came back up from the toilets. I wasn't using then. I was clean then, came back and he said, 'Oh babe, can I have a seat? I feel a bit funny'. I said, 'Alright, sit here'. I've got my one-year-old son with me at the time, our son. I'm sitting talking to him and I'm getting no response. His head is on my lap. The next time I look, he's just blue. No one would help. It was in the middle of Newcastle city centre. No one would help him. There was a doctor in the crowd. When I was screaming for help, obviously

	a crowd came fucking running. There was a doctor, and he wouldn't touch him.
FD:	Why not?
B:	He's a junkie.
FD:	What did he say?
B:	'I can't treat him. I can't do anything'. I had to revive him, not forgetting that I've got my son in the pram. Give him CPR. Luckily, I was a first aider, and I knew what I was doing. I had him breathing by the time the ambulance came. He was physically dead on my lap.

In this distressing account, Beckie's partner nearly died in her lap. She experiences this stigmatising event as deadly, as (almost) killing him. She is clear that 'no one would help him', not even a doctor, because he was a 'junkie'. Stratified by this identity, all his other identities ceased to matter. He was not seen as a father or partner, even with Beckie and their baby by his side. He could not even be a patient. Beckie notes that the doctor 'wouldn't touch him'. She is pointing here to the way the 'junkie' figure is connected to notions of disease and contagion. It was the skin-to-skin intimacy that the doctor and crowd were refusing. They would look – 'obviously a crowd came fucking running' – but they would not touch him. Due to this stratification, he was constrained in the most extreme way: almost dying.

In the next account, a participant called Lucy is forced to leave a party due to an 'addict' or 'junkie' identity that puts her under suspicion of criminality. Unlike other party guests under the same circumstance of a missing purse, this stratification as an 'addict' – 'because of the association', as she puts it – immediately turned her into a thief, to the point that she felt unable to stay:

> The stigma can actually be horrible, because, let me give you an example. There was a party and me and my boyfriend were *known*, and somebody couldn't find their purse and they went in my bag three times, ranting and raving, and then they found it in their car. So that part of it is really insulting. Because they presume you're a thief all the time. And it really made me upset, and I was really angry. I wouldn't steal off people. And it was a big family event on my boyfriend's side and his mum was stressed and there was loads of politics going on. But because of the association, because they know of our lifestyle, they ... there was this panic and I remember just being so angry, I thought for fuck's sake, you've already been through my bag once, the accusation is such an insult ... Then this person just rang up and said 'oh, I found my purse', and I just thought where's your bloody apology. And I just remember storming out and I remember just feeling so angry. I was so angry and so humiliated. Because there was this person ranting and

raving around this place, and the image of ... everyone was asked, but me and my boyfriend were asked too much, too intently, to the point that I just wanted to go, and I felt really tearful and ... God, the insults I've had to take.

In Lucy's 'association' with drugs and addiction, she is connected and stratified by images of deviance and criminality. Under a situation of pressure, these often-invisible structures are voiced and publicly made known in a most explosive and humiliating way. Unlike others at the party, Lucy and her partner are accused and questioned 'too much, too intently', signalling them out as Other. Feeling humiliated, angry, tearful, and ultimately unwelcome, they leave.

Trying to explain further about how this stratification works, this time, in relation to the 'addict' as 'diseased' (like Beckie's example), Lucy recounts another pressurised incident in which her boyfriend 'was wacked around the face by his step-mum and we were told that we should have labels put on us saying that we are dirty junkies':

There was a lot of politics going on because, basically, we were using [drugs] and we were in a stage of moving house, and there was a lot of our stuff kept in their garden. But this box, where our needles were, were in this bag, really deep, and his father must have really gone in his cupboard and really gone to find them. So, he made this big deal about finding these pins in this box and then, they'd had a kid, and the boy wasn't very well, and I just remember the woman came storming through this kitchen and just wacked him. And she was American. And she was just screaming at us, saying you 'fucking junkies, you should wear a label, you don't bring that shit [into our house]'.

The syringes ('pins') here are key to this story and how this stratification works. As Nicole Vitellone (2010) explains in her work on the 'sociology of the syringe', syringes are already 'designated disgusting'; they are connected to images of disease and contamination. The pins become the catalyst of this outburst. Speaking directly to the invisibility of how this disease imagery and stratification works, the stepmother says that Lucy and her partner should wear a label, marking them out as 'junkies'. With this, we are reminded of the original meaning of the word stigma rooted in Ancient Greek to denote a bodily sign: '[T]he term stigma ... refer[s] to bodily signs designed to expose something unusual and bad about the moral status of the signifier' (Goffman, 1963, 1). In her recent book, Tyler (2020) traces examples of stigma as derived from the root 'stig-', meaning to prick or to puncture, from ancient penal tattooing, to the marking of slaves, to the ways Jewish people were exhibited with cardboard signs saying 'I have been excluded from the national community' during anti-Jewish pogroms, and to the modern-day use of shaming techniques in the US where convicted petty criminals are forced to hold placards or wear billboards outside shopping malls stating 'I am a thief' (Tyler, 2020, 145). In her rage, then, the stepmother is drawing on a long and violent history of the use of physical signs and markers to denote body-persons as bad and otherwise subhuman. In these two accounts, Lucy and her partner lose their identities as guests, as family members, as they become stratified and blocked by this 'junkie' identity as criminal and diseased.

The third account of stigma I want to share is from Tina. Tina tells me about a horrific experience in which she is stratified as an 'addict' and prostitute, and shamed and blocked from being able to work – even though she had done all the training. She explains how she calls the recruitment agency about her criminal record and is invited into their offices to show them her Disclosure and Barring Service (DBS) check. Her DBS shows multiple old charges – 'these are all years ago' – for soliciting sex and drug possession:

> Me, like an idiot, phoned her up [the recruiter] and said, 'I don't know if you'll take me on with my record'. She said, 'bring it [the DBS check] in, you'll be alright'. I took it in, she went downstairs, said she'd gone to see the manager, and whilst she was downstairs, women kept on coming up and looking at me. There was a room downstairs with women all on computers and they kept coming up and pretending, asking questions to the girl, then the two managers came up, called me into the back room, she said we're sorry but even if we send this to head office, they'll say no. So, I said okay and just walked out. I was angry, but I didn't show it. I should have got them done for the way I was treated. And I'd done all the training and everything. I had to go all the way to bloody East London, you know, borrow money to get the bus fare up there every day. And then they told me no. And that put me off trying again ... All I wanted was a job. And it's not good work care work. It's only £6 an hour. I just wanted to do something, you know, to feel good inside, instead of feeling dirty all the time. It just fucking makes you feel like, fuck it.

The DBS check continues to mark Tina out – stratifying her as an addict and prostitute even though she no longer uses drugs or solicits sex. It is an identity that continues to follow her, to define and restrict her. We are alerted again to this feeling of shame and dirtiness that is often felt in these processes of stratification, what Zigon (2019, 53) discusses as 'the addict' as akin to shit. She is left feeling dirty by this experience and questions the point of giving up drugs if she continues to be stratified by them in these most life-constraining ways.

In all three examples, then, it is not the person's addiction that is causing these restrictions to life, but their connection to these stratifying identities. It is not the drug or addiction that nearly kills Beckie's partner, but its association with contagion that means a doctor will not treat him. It is not Lucy's drug use that drives her to leave a party, but the fact that she is labelled and accused of being a thief. The same goes for Tina. It is not her past dependency that means she cannot work, but her DBS record that continues to mark her out in this way as Other, turning her into an object of ridicule and entertainment for a sniggering recruitment agency.

Having seen the way stigma operates through these networks and always in process as a means of blocking life chances and what people can become, I want to return to this idea that, where bad connections are happening, good ones are also possible. Key to this is what Peta Malins (2004) wrote (see previous section): *if we allow it*. Therefore, opening up space for people who use drugs to exist differently, outside of the confines of addiction, involves us all.

Making space for being otherwise: in solidarity with people who use drugs

Our role, then, as sociological researchers of health and illness, if we want to act in solidarity with people who use drugs and try to reduce these stigmatising events, is to see these lives as worthy lives. In Latimer's (2018, 833) essay on dementia stigma, she explores the ageing body, which much like the addicted body, 'can be experienced as disgusting and repulsive because it represents deviation from what is most cherished in modernity and contemporary preoccupations with specific forms of personhood'. Latimer argues that, by researching closely with stigmatised groups, or 'dwelling alongside', as she puts it, we can see worlds differently together. Latimer emphasises the livingness in those otherwise stigmatised lives and says that they can instead be seen as 'a possible way to resist the dominant forms of personhood mobilized in late modern capitalism and which "others" those no longer willing or able to be response-able and fold themselves into its demands' (Latimer, 2018, 849). For example, in my research over the last fifteen years or so, I have been struck by the complex, generative ways people make their lives *with* drugs. In a recent essay, a colleague and I reflect on the life of Kim, a fifty-something Black British woman who is adamant that she will continue smoking crack cocaine until the day she dies:

> If I went into old age and I was still smoking cocaine, I'd be a soldier ... I'd be a toughie, I'd be a real toughie. I'd be really proud of myself that I hadn't bowed to social pressure – treatment and this and that and

police … Personally, I'd like to use until the day I die and that would be my choice. (Dennis and Pienaar, 2023, 796).

Kim refuses treatment narratives that erase the life-affirming aspects of her drug use and seek her 'recovery'. Even though her drug use may be judged as dependent and therefore problematic by outsiders, she tells us how she cares for herself and others. Like many other people I have met who use drugs in ways that attract the label of dependency and addiction, she refuses a narrative that she is ill. Instead, if listened to, she is changing the terms of what it means to live a worthwhile life.

To drive home what is at stake here, if this is not already clear from these harrowing accounts of blocked, constrained lives, every year for a decade now, more people in the UK are dying of 'drug-related' causes. In an article published in 2021, I argued that we are failing to respond to the needs of people who use drugs, particularly through our abstinence-driven treatment system, where, as we see in James' testimony, this does not work for everyone. Rather than doubling down on drugs as 'the problem' and therefore the solution being abstinence, James is encouraging us to see the problem as coming from elsewhere. Here, I have located this 'problem' in a process of stratification that is dramatised in the three accounts of blocked becoming, with the first example showing explicitly how life can be ended by these processes. As we have seen, it is not the drug that is responsible for these constraints, but its connections to those images, knowledges, and objects (such as the 'pins' in Lucy's story) that depict these person-bodies as 'addicts' – diseased, devoid, less-than-human, or, in Latimer's (2018) terms, a living death. To intervene and undo these 'blockages', we must learn to dwell alongside these body-persons differently, work to become more response-able to them, and in essence, value these lives as worthy lives.

Let me now give an example of what I mean. After publishing the article saying that rising drug-related deaths were linked to our limited response-ability to these lives, particularly when it comes to prescribing diamorphine, I received several desperate emails from people who use drugs, their family members, and a prescriber. They all spoke of how their lives or the lives of their loved ones or people they worked with had been made on substances such as diamorphine (not despite them) – a family, career, home-life, their health and wellbeing – and these were now under threat as they had been told their prescription would be stopped or had already been.

One woman wrote to me explaining how she had been on a daily pickup prescription of diamorphine since 1992, 'working, feeling fine, healthy, exercising, et cetera' until her prescription was recently and abruptly ended. She felt forced back to the illicit market and now has non-healing wounds from her injecting sites. She has begged to be restarted on diamorphine, but was told this is not possible. One daughter who writes to me on behalf of her father struggles to understand how medical professionals are failing to see the good that diamorphine has done in her father's life – allowing him to work, care for his children, grandchildren, and manage back pain and other chronic health issues – and cannot 'fathom how any medical professional would hold themselves accountable to make a decision to stop it!'

To challenge stigma as a relational process of becoming blocked and act in solidarity with people who use drugs, we must open ourselves up to these different ways of being and question where harm or the problem of drug use is actually coming from. As Latimer (2018, 846) puts it in relation to people with dementia who are often described as 'away' and elsewhere, 'we have to consider that it may be "us" that are elsewhere. Us, with our projects and our futures who are really "away"'. By seeing stigma as relational in the processes of blocked becoming – nearly dying, unable to socialise, unemployed – rather than the consequences of the drug or addiction, we can shift an image of addiction as inevitable decline and harm. To reiterate from the epigraph: 'By shifting our relations to the characteristics we are being made to see as [the disease problem/addiction], we can refigure them as ways of being in the world differently, and as such, as other ways of being human' (Latimer, 2018, 848).

As researchers, we must tell such counter-stories and spotlight grassroots movements where alternative ways of living with drugs are taking place, like in James' experience of harm reduction activism. As Zigon (2019, 111) explains, 'to practice harm reduction is to let-users-be and to build worlds that are open to this letting-be'. This is an alternative form of care that refuses the 'negative imagery of the addict' that 'result[s] in the fact that the only kind of care available for the "addict", when any care is available at all, is that biopolitical care that demands that the "addict" becomes "clean"' (Zigon, 2019, 141). I would add that this is different, too, from the biomedical care predicated on the 'addicted subject' accepting their status as 'sick', a logic that anti-stigma work frequently relies on. Therefore, in these alternative acts of care and solidarity, we make space for the kinds of being-with drugs that James and Kim call for in questioning where 'the problem' is coming from and our role in this problem-making. In other words, it is through these acts of care that we can foster acceptance and dismantle stigma.

Conclusion

In this chapter, I have presented three accounts of stigma as 'blocked becomings', where people who use drugs have been prevented from becoming a patient, guest, and employee, as well as many other identities such as partner, son, and father. Rather than thinking of stigma as something that happens prior to these events – as a belief system 'out there' and already stigmatised individuals entering the event – I have examined the ways in which stigma materialises in these events as constricting peoples' capacities to act and be outside of the addict identity. The blocking effects often attributed to the drug, addiction, or the failed person – depicted here through accounts of near-fatal overdose, social and familial exclusion, and unemployment – are coming from these processes. In this sense, more so than in Goffman's (1963) classic account of stigma as relational, attention is steered away from the individual or aggregates of individuals to that of the relation. In doing so, this also does something else. Instead of looking to anti-stigma work that claims to tackle stigmatising beliefs, this approach invites a closer look at where the problem is coming from.

By attuning to the complex interplays between 'the social' and 'the individual', this is not about seeing the human behind the illness as anti-addiction stigma campaigns proclaim: '[Stigmatising beliefs and attitudes] create stereotypes, judgements and biases, stopping us from seeing the human being behind the illness' (NHS Addiction Provider Alliance, 2022). But rather, this is precisely about seeing the human in the illness or, even more precisely, seeing the human because these practices are no longer seen as illness. But there is more. By becoming response-able to people's lives with drugs as alternative modes of living or being human, we can ask more productive questions to the effect of what more we can do to enable flourishing with drugs, rather than simply how we make people end and recover from them. It is this socio-material care work that I think of as anti-stigma work.

Could things be different?

- It is rarely helpful to understand frequent drug use as addiction. Stigma could be reduced by developing greater acceptance of different ways of living with drugs.
- If frequent, heavy drug use was not always seen as a problem of addiction that needs to be reversed, people might be enabled (and resources allocated) to live with drugs in more positive ways.
- If this is going to be achieved, then people working in these fields need to collaborate with affected communities and particularly activists who are already involved in this work of reconceptualising and putting into practice alternative care structures.
- More training and research informed by the harm reduction movement and ethos will be needed to undo dominant thinking about regular drug use and promote more creative thinking about the diverse role of drugs in peoples' lives.

Acknowledgements

Thank you to the editors for producing such a warm and generative space for collaboration on this project. I am especially thankful to Oli Williams and Amy Chandler for their insightful and constructive comments on the chapter, and to Andy Guise for his thoughts on an earlier draft.

References

Addison, M., McGovern, W. and McGovern, R. (2022) *Drugs, Identity and Stigma*, Basingstoke: Palgrave Macmillan.

Alexandrescu, L. (forthcoming) *Drugscapes: Imaginaries of Intoxication, Dependency, and Control*, London: Routledge.

BBC Radio 4 (2022) 'High anxiety: The deadly trade in street Valium', *BBC*, [online] 6 November 2022, Available from: https://www.bbc.co.uk/programmes/m001dnbr [Accessed 7 June 2024].

Campbell, N. (2023) 'Confronting the drug war session 5: Deconstructing the brain disease model of addiction', *YouTube*, [online] 3 August, Available from: https://www.youtube.com/watch?v=qvovM4eF7d8 [Accessed 7 June 2024].

Deleuze, G. and Guattari, F. (1987) *A Thousand Plateaus: Capitalism and Schizophrenia*, Minneapolis, MN: University of Minnesota Press.

Dennis, F. (2021) 'Advocating for diamorphine: Cosmopolitical care and collective action in the ruins of the "old British system"', *Critical Public Health*, 31(2): 144–55.

Dennis, F. and Pienaar, K. (2023) 'Refusing recovery, living a "wayward life": A feminist analysis of women's drug use', *The Sociological Review* 71(4): 781–800.

Fraser, S., Pienaar, K., Dilkes-Frayne, E., Moore, D., Kokanovic, R., Treloar, C. and Dunlop, A. (2017) 'Addiction stigma and the biopolitics of liberal modernity: A qualitative analysis', *International Journal of Drug Policy* 44: 192–201.

Goffman, E. (1963) *Stigma: Notes on the Management of Spoiled Identity*, Harmondsworth and Ringwood: Penguin.

Hannem, S. and Brucket, C. (2012) *Stigma Revisited: Implications of the Mark*, Ottawa: University of Ottawa Press.

Harris, M., Guy, D., Picchio, C.A., White, T.M., Rhodes, T. and Lazarus, J.V. (2021) 'Conceptualising hepatitis C stigma: A thematic synthesis of qualitative research', *International Journal of Drug Policy*, 96: 103320.

Kulesza, M., Larimer, M. and Rao, D. (2013) 'Substance use related stigma: What we know and the way forward', *Journal of Addictive Behaviours, Therapy and Rehabilitation*, 2(2): 782.

Latimer, J. (2018) 'Repelling neoliberal world-making? How the ageing–dementia relation is reassembling the social', *The Sociological Review*, 66(4): 832–56.

Malins, P. (2004) 'Machinic assemblages: Deleuze, Guattari and an ethico-aesthetics of drug use', *Janus Head*, 7(1): 84–104.

NHS Addiction Provider Alliance (2022) 'Stigma kills campaign', *NHS*, [online], Available from: https://www.nhsapa.org/stigma [Accessed 7 June 2024].

Parker, R. and Aggleton, P. (2003) 'HIV and AIDS-related stigma and discrimination: A conceptual framework and implications for action', *Social Science and Medicine*, 57(1): 13–24.

Paton, K. (2018) 'Beyond legacy: Backstage stigmatisation and "trickle-up" politics of urban regeneration', *The Sociological Review*, 66(4): 919–34.

Radcliffe, P. and Stevens, A. (2008) 'Are drug treatment services only for "thieving junkie scumbags"? Drug users and the management of stigmatised identities', *Social Science and Medicine*, 67(7): 1065–73.

Scambler, G. (2018) 'Heaping blame on shame: "Weaponising stigma" for neoliberal times', *The Sociological Review*, 66(4): 766–82.

Simmonds, L. and Coomber, R. (2009) 'Injecting drug users: A stigmatised and stigmatising population', *International Journal of Drug Policy*, 20(2): 121–30.

Tyler, I. (2018) 'Resituating Erving Goffman: From stigma power to Black power', *The Sociological Review*, 66(4): 744–65.

Tyler, I. (2020) *Stigma: The Machinery of Inequality*, London: Bloomsbury Publishing.

Tyler, I. and Slater, T. (2018) *The Sociology of Stigma*, London: SAGE/Sociological Review Monograph.

Vitellone, N. (2010) 'Just another night in the shooting gallery? The syringe, space, and affect', *Environment and Planning D: Society and Space*, 28(5): 867–80.

Zigon, J. (2019) *A War on People: Drug User Politics and a New Ethics of Community*, Oakland: University of California Press.

8

How Stigma Emerges and Mutates: The Case of Long COVID Stigma

Hannah Farrimond and Mike Michael

Introduction

How do new stigmas emerge? How do they relate to existing stigma? Why are we seeing an emergent devaluation and discrimination of people who have long COVID, given how common it is to have experienced COVID-19? This chapter explores these questions using the 'stigma mutation' theory that I (HF) have proposed elsewhere (Farrimond, 2021). Stigma mutation theory suggests that the emergence of stigma, and how stigma changes over time, can be understood along three dimensions: 'lineage' (how stigma is linked to other stigmas and histories of stigma); 'variation' (how stigma changes emerge in relation to differing environments and cultures); and 'strength' (how stigma can intensify or weaken over time). In this chapter, we propose an extension of this theory by suggesting that these dimensions are interrelated; stigmas constitute a dynamic 'assemblage' of connections which are both predictable (what we call 'territorialised') and unpredictable and disrupted (what we call 'de-territorialised'). In other words, there are multiple relations of connections gathering to form and reform stigmas. Some are expected, given what we know about the persistence of stigma, while others are unexpected, creating complex new effects.

To explore the usefulness of this theorisation, we explain how and why long COVID stigma (Pantelic et al, 2022) has come about. We suggest long COVID stigma shows clear continuity with existing stigmas related to chronic illness, gender, poverty, State dependence, and inactivity in neo-capitalist societies. Simultaneously, long COVID stigma is being de-territorialised (or disrupted) in a multiplicity of ways, for example, by activists and unpredictable events. We also consider the symbolic value of any given stigma. For instance, long COVID stigma may be amplified in the face of a collective desire to forget COVID-19, yet stigma may also lessen via active resistance and/or cultural change.

How and why stigma mutates

We start out with a definition of stigma as the holding of a derogated social identity (Goffman, 1963). Importantly, though, this devalued status is produced through complex processes, both interpersonal and sociocultural, which change over time. The original 'stigma mutation' theory was developed during the first two years of the COVID-19 pandemic (2020–22). Here, it seemed, was the perfect example through which to consider stigma emergence. COVID-19 was a completely novel disease, and the pandemic was something for which the world (or our corner of it in the UK) was unprepared. Any stigma attached to it, therefore, was also new. COVID-19 stigma emerged and developed in real-time. From its inception, the Western reporting of its origins as 'Chinese' bore the hallmarks of racism (Choi, 2021; Gui, 2021). Viruses, especially highly contagious ones with a death rate beyond expectations, are also greatly feared; fear and risk are core drivers of stigma (Jones et al, 1984).

It was no surprise, therefore, that with the pandemic of COVID-19 came COVID-19 stigma, although in complex, divergent, and sometimes unpredictable ways. As much as it emerged viciously in some settings and towards some groups (Bagcchi, 2020; Roelen et al, 2020), it quickly dissipated in other situations. Indeed, declaring one's COVID-19 status online became somewhat commonplace in the celebrity world. Nevertheless, shame and blame abounded. Such stigma was driven partly by the desire to identify who was contaminated, but was also 'weaponised' (Scambler, 2018) – that is, individuals were held responsible for their own infection, which conveniently pointed the spotlight away from structural failures by government, such as a lack of pandemic preparedness (Cooper et al, 2023).

The holding of a stigmatised social identity is always complicated. Indeed, part of the stress for stigmatised individuals is the uncertainty surrounding social interactions (Goffman, 1963). More recent sociological rethinking has emphasised that the labelling and stereotyping of 'others' is an ideological matter (Link and Phelan, 2001; Tyler and Slater, 2018; Tyler, 2020). In other words, the creation of 'others' is often beneficial to those in power – structurally and institutionally. Scambler (2018) uses the example of how neoliberal governments perpetuate stigmatising individualistic discourses that frame those living in poverty, dependent on State funds, and/or disabled or sick as blameworthy for their own predicament. The theory of 'stigma mutation' is situated within this work, with its emphasis on power, process, and history. It aims to add depth to thinking not only about continuity (for example, with past stigmas), but also discontinuity and change. From this perspective, stigma is both produced by, and mutates from, the actions of the powerful in line with their needs, but also reflects wider cultural resonances. It is, thus, both *top-down* and *bottom-up*.

Having COVID-19 today is not a matter of shame and blame in the same way that it was in 2020. Furthermore, new forms of stigma, such as long COVID stigma, are emerging. How can we account for these ebbs and flows in stigma presentation, discourse, and behaviours? In the next section, we examine each of the three dimensions of stigma mutation suggested in the original theory: 1) lineage, 2) variation, and 3) strength. We explore each dimension in relation to long COVID stigma. As such, this chapter represents an extension of the case study of COVID-19 stigma, and also leads us to reflect critically on how we might conceptualise change over time, which is complex and multifaceted. To this end, we draw on post actor-network theory and assemblage theory (Deleuze and Guattari, 1988; Mol, 2002; Latour, 2005, 2010; Michael, 2017) as a means of further nuancing stigma mutation. To be clear, this is a theoretical reading. There is not (yet) a whole heap of empirical evidence in relation to long COVID stigma, although that might change.

Long COVID and its stigmatisation

Long COVID is the name given to the symptoms of COVID-19 that persist beyond the initial days and weeks of the illness. There is no one definition of it. It is usually taken to mean ongoing symptoms after three months of initial illness (Chaichana et al, 2023). We are using long COVID as the current popular and scientific definition, and one originally defined by an international movement of patients (Perego et al, 2020; Callard and Perego, 2021).

Long COVID is extremely common, with up to 65 million sufferers worldwide, but it is also acutely neglected within healthcare (The Lancet, 2023). One of the core conundrums is the causal mechanisms of long COVID. A recent review identified several potential causes, such as immune problems, disruptions to the microbiota, clotting problems, dysfunctional neurological signalling, and psychological factors (Davis et al, 2023). This, in turn, has raised questions over how similar long COVID is to other disorders, such as post-viral fatigue, myalgic encephalomyelitis (ME)/chronic fatigue syndrome (CFS), and postural tachycardia syndrome (PoTS), among others. This similarity/dissimilarity has become a site of huge contention, particularly when it comes to considering whether long COVID should be designated as primarily biological or psychological in origin.

Professor Paul Garner's (2021) account of recovering from long COVID in the *British Medical Journal*, through, in his words, moving on from a purely biomedical account, and resetting his dysfunctional autonomic neural patterns (that is, his 'thinking'), caused uproar within the chronic illness community. This was because they perceived this as a rejection of their long struggle to have ME/CFS recognised as a biological (and not psychological) disorder. This 'psychiatrisation' of conditions such as ME (and now, we suggest, long COVID) is perceived by those within the community as a denial of their lived experience, and thus as a form of 'epistemic injustice' that can lead to unwanted or inappropriate treatments (Spandler and Allen, 2018). Despite controversies over the causes of long COVID, what is not in doubt is the awful experience of having it; 'long-haulers' can experience increased risk of heart attack and stroke, multi-organ problems, neurological damage, extreme 'brain fog', and fatigue months or years after initial infection (Davis et al, 2023).

Given the lack of consensus over long COVID as a scientific entity, we suggest that long COVID is best thought of in terms of 'multiple ontologies' (Mol, 2002). By this, we mean it is enacted through, and composed of, different and diverse arrays of practices, discourses, technologies, and objects. Each of these arrays comprises an ontology – a version of long COVID that is made and remade by different people and communities that can entail different forms of expert knowledge and skill and/or different types of lay experience. Following Mol, we see these ontologies as interacting in various ways – sometimes in synergy, sometimes in parallel, and sometimes in opposition. We can address the patterns of interaction by drawing on the notion of assemblages, which, put simply, are variously configured patterns of different elements and their interrelations (Deleuze and Guattari, 1988). Each entity itself comprises an assemblage, that is, a pattern of relations and elements (Latour, 2005, 2010) and, for present purposes, can be thought of as an ontology (Mol, 2002).

In the work of Deleuze and Guattari, these associations are understood in relation to plant structures. Patterns can be structured and routinised (or territorialised or striated) or they become fluid and unpredictable (de-territorialised or smooth). The structured, territorialised patterns are similar to roots which anchor plants, such as trees; the fluid, de-territorialised patterns are similar to 'rhizomes', which are networks of plant matter that can shoot off in unpredictable ways from their nodes underground. Each element in an assemblage can interrelate with any other element. Hence, elements that might seem distant in space and time, materially and culturally, can become close, and vice versa. We might say, therefore, that the assemblage is topological; the patterns can be reformed in many ways, but hold together as an entity.

What, then, are the implications of the multiple forms of long COVID for any stigma attached to it? At a general level, our reason for applying this assemblage framework is that it adds an additional dimension to 'stigma mutation' theory. If, broadly speaking, 'stigma mutation' theory hints at a broader model of evolution in which particular stigmatisations come to prominence because of their increasingly better 'fit' into their heterogeneous environment, assemblage theory interjects a process of 'involution'. Here, involution implies unpredictability whereby unexpected elements can enter into a process of stigmatisation, or exit it, in ways that can change the environment and, thereby, the meaning of 'fit' (Ansell Pearson, 1999).

As we shall also argue, this allows us to explore how better to articulate and operationalise the dimensions of 'lineage', 'variation', and 'strength'. In relation to the specificities of long COVID stigmatisations, this means that we become sensitised to how these are heterogeneously constituted, exist in relation to multiple ontologies that interact and intersect in different patterns, and are emergent/changing. It further suggests that a methodologically diverse approach is needed to study long COVID stigma; we need to engage with different types of data. After all, long COVID stigma might be enacted in conversations with friends and families, family care practitioner records or referrals, human resources guidelines, the national media, social media comments, government statements, and scientific repositories – and these might interrelate in multiple ways. The analysis we offer in this chapter, thus, needs to be treated as highly contingent, given that neither long COVID, nor long COVID stigma, are reified or fixed either scientifically or socially at any given time.

Perhaps naively, given that I (HF) have experienced post-viral fatigue after COVID-19 myself and that I had written about COVID-19 stigma, I did not automatically think of long COVID in terms of generating stigma. My own experience of having post-viral fatigue after COVID-19 was that my friends and family were sympathetic and that many could relate. I was not the only one to 'feel shit' after COVID-19. My friends also had other friends who had severe long COVID. Again, this seemed to be a matter of sympathy as well as slight bewilderment at COVID-19 as a disease: what type of thing was this that took down previously healthy young(ish) scholars, writers, people who went running, who worked out?

Work was another matter. I quickly learned that 'recovery' was the narrative required there. That should have been the clue. Narratives about long COVID were diverging, and negative talk about those with long COVID was emerging. Within the media, articles with titles such as 'The stigma of long COVID: Why don't people believe it's real' (Lindsay, 2022) appeared. Public comments on an article in the UK's *Daily Mail* reporting that one in five people were unable to return to work a year after COVID-19 infection contained pejorative attributions galore: 'Long Covid is just ME'; 'Long Covid is the new bad back'; 'the new fibromyalgia'; 'young people lack resilience' (Morrison, 2023). Attributions of laziness, lack of legitimacy as a disease, and malingering were emerging. It was later revealed that the then UK Prime Minister, Boris Johnson, had written one word on a report on long COVID in 2020: 'Bollocks'. On Twitter, it was suggested that some celebrities and influencers were hiding their long COVID status, fearful of devaluing their healthy brand. Others used 'before' and 'after' photos to show the devastating impact long COVID had on them, such as on social media on the newly inaugurated #LongCovidAwarenessDay.

Long COVID stigma was also emerging as the object of research. Pantelic and colleagues identified two main types: 1) institutional stigma (discrimination), in terms of being ignored and disbelieved by healthcare professionals; and 2) internalised stigma, in terms of feeling devalued, guilty, and shameful as a person about still being ill with long COVID (Pantelic and Alwan, 2021; Pantelic et al, 2022). Subsequently, Pantelic and colleagues have developed a 13-item survey scale which adds a third dimension: 'anticipated' stigma (anticipating bias/poor treatment by others). Their initial findings using the scale were astonishing, with 95 per cent of the sample reporting some experience of stigma (sometimes/often/always), and 76 per cent reporting it as a frequent occurrence (often/always). Interestingly, those with clinical diagnoses of long COVID experienced more stigma than those without. Perhaps those with a formal diagnosis were more severely ill, so hiding their status was not an option. It does suggest, however, that gaining a medical diagnosis is not acting as a method of legitimation, and thus of stigma relief.

International scholars have identified similar stigma among those with long COVID in Canada (Damant et al, 2023). The 'Post COVID-19 Condition Stigma Questionnaire' suggests that those who were disabled/not employed scored the highest for stigma, which was also associated with depression, anxiety, and severity. A qualitative review of the small amount of interview studies with long COVID patients (MacPherson et al, 2022) found that participants reported discordance between their knowledge and that of others such as family or healthcare professionals (for example, expecting it to have resolved much faster). This, in turn, led to feelings of stigma, both internalised shame and blame and anticipatory fear of judgement.

In summary, research, alongside wider media sources, are identifying the prevalence and lived realities of long COVID stigma. However, its nuances have yet to be explored. Little work to date has identified why long COVID has been stigmatised so quickly. COVID-19 stigma itself has lessened over time, while long COVID stigma is being amplified. We suggest, then, that although COVID-19 and long COVID stigmas are related, they also differ across key dimensions. Although long COVID has been recognised (and thus legitimated) by medical authorities such as the World Health Organization (2022), there are features – such as uncertain aetiology (causation) and existing negative narratives around chronic illness – that are causing problems for its bearers. We return, then, to the idea of long COVID as emergent sets of knowledges (ontologies) that are at once pulled together (and contested) within an assemblage as a starting point to understand how stigmatisation is manifested. Such processes are complex, and unstable, but, at times, also follow well-worn grooves (for example, drawing on prior stigma and prejudice against certain groups). In other words, stigmatisation is at once territorialised (predictable) and de-territorialised (unpredictable) but, as we shall argue, certain patterns of long COVID stigma are nevertheless detectable.

On the emergence of long COVID stigmatisation

In this section, we examine the emergence of long COVID stigma according to each of the three dimensions of 'stigma mutation' defined in the original theory: 1) lineage, 2) variation, and 3) strength. We explore how each might be understood in relation to the dynamics of a long COVID stigmatisation assemblage.

Stigma lineage

Recent contributions on the sociology of stigma highlight the importance of history for understanding stigma at the structural/institutional level (Tyler, 2020). The term 'lineage' used here refers to evolutionary heritage. In relation to stigma, this refers to its predecessors and relations with other stigmas. In the context of long COVID stigma, there are some obvious predecessors. One is the stigma of COVID-19 itself. COVID-19 is part of a long line of feared contagious diseases, including but not limited to Ebola, SARS (severe acute respiratory syndrome), MERS (Middle East respiratory syndrome), and HIV, and, going back in time, other 'plagues' such as the Great (bubonic) Plague, cholera, and leprosy. Such contagious diseases are feared due to their risk of illness and death. However, as Strong (1990) has argued, this quickly turns into fear of the diseased 'other', groups, or individuals who are perceived not only as carriers in the biological sense, but to blame in a moral sense for spreading the disease.

This blame and shame come from many sources. For example, the amplification of anti-Chinese/Asian stigma was marked across the world, identifying China/Asia as a common source of deadly viruses (Darling-Hammond et al, 2020). This was then amplified in the political sphere by Donald Trump (then President of the US) using negative language such as 'Kung Flu'. The stigmatisation of COVID-19 has been complex and has changed over time (for example, it is less potent now than in March 2020), but it is hardly surprising that a disorder that emerges out of a stigmatised disease itself holds the potential for stigmatisation, but for different reasons.

A second predecessor for long COVID stigma is the stigmatisation of other post-viral syndromes. The link between the ongoing symptoms of long COVID and other chronic illnesses, particularly ME/CFS and PoTS, was made early on, and debate continues as to their precise relationship (for example, is long COVID, after a certain period, better referred to as ME?) (Davis et al, 2023). There is a large body of sociological and anthropological work that has articulated the stigmatisation of 'liminal' illnesses, namely, those that are often invisible, fluctuating, and without definitive diagnostic tests. 'Liminality' is very well described by Jackson (2008, 332) in their articulation of the 'mind–body' borderlands of chronic pain, claiming that features of it 'result in the perception of sufferers as transgressing the categorical divisions between mind and body and as confounding the codes of morality surrounding sickness and health, turning them into liminal creatures, whose ontological status provokes stigmatised reactions in others'. Such dualism, which itself pulls on the stigma of mental illness as less valid than physical illness, is inherent in the stigmatisation of long COVID predecessors such as ME (Froelich et al, 2022). Their designation (by some) as *all in the mind* is positioned as an act of disbelief in the legitimacy of the disorders as biological entities. Furthermore, their status as *functional* implies that such illnesses should primarily be treated by psychological means (for example, with cognitive behavioural therapy) rather than biologically. Ballering et al (2021) have suggested that this dualist thinking (biological versus psychological) also underlies long COVID stigma.

A final aspect of long COVID stigma lineage is the stigma of respiratory disease (Carel, 2024). As a recent opinion piece suggests, stigma is the missing piece of the treatment jigsaw in chronic obstructive pulmonary disease (COPD) and other respiratory conditions, sometimes unwittingly perpetuated by those in healthcare themselves (Mathioudakis et al, 2021). Smokers, in particular, are demonised and held responsible for their respiratory issues, though this is also because their 'pollution' is understood to affect others (Farrimond and Joffe, 2006). Long COVID (as implicating and extending the respiratory issues of COVID-19) is, thus, not exempt from this lineage of existing stigmatisation, emerging within a trajectory of already 'orphaned' disorders that attract societal blame and institutional underfunding.

It is clear, therefore, that long COVID stigma fits within multiple lineages, both of novel COVID-19 stigma and already existing stigmas of disease and disadvantage. Within an assemblage, we can consider this lineage as 'territorialised' elements, in other words, associations which are strong, well-established, often occupying well-worn grooves of discrimination and disadvantage. In the case of long COVID, this raises questions about whether it is helpful, hindering, or 'piggy-backing' to co-opt those in ME clinical and lay communities to the long COVID cause. It could be argued that there is strength in numbers. Equally, by being co-opted into the liminal illness category of 'medically unexplained symptoms', long COVID has experienced stigma transfer, rehearsing already well-worn debates concerning whether these disorders are *all in the mind*, biological, or something else. Conversely, we also need to be alert to the possibility that long COVID's (still) disputed status might benefit from alliance with other chronic illness networks through a renewed interest in post-viral fatigue – as a form of de-territorialisation that might challenge existing stigma lineages.

A further intersection with other stigma occurs around the consequences of long COVID and their political framing. One effect of long COVID, like the other liminal illnesses, is that people are no longer able to work, making them less productive economically. Consequently, dependence on State support (welfare benefits) is also increased. Scambler (2018) has argued that within neoliberal capitalist culture, stigma has been 'weaponised'. The shame of being poor or using State benefits has been used by the ruling elites as a discourse to allocate blame, holding these groups responsible for their own plight through attributions of out-of-control behaviour, unhealthiness, and laziness, as inadequate citizens. This pairing of shame with blame conveniently draws attention away from the political causes of poverty and disability, such as structural inequality. Within this narrative, the public is divided into 'taxpayers' and 'scroungers', the latter representing a net loss to prudent management of the economy (Clarke, 1997).

Long COVID stigma makes sense within these existing political lineages of devaluation; attributions of laziness or using benefits rather than working have, for example, appeared on social media. Once more, we see a highly entrenched territorialisation in play. Equally, COVID-19's impact on work practices and the discourses of wellbeing can also be understood as an example of 'de-territorialisation', where new possibilities for alternative understandings concerning living with chronic illness, and thus long COVID, are potentially opened up (for example, through the high numbers of people affected).

To conclude this section, lineage is, thus, 'fundamental to understanding new stigma mutation ... identifying the anchors of stigma helps make sense of its present forms' (Farrimond, 2021, 174). It is important to stress, however, that even within existing histories of stigma, this does not mean that devaluation is inevitable, or that such histories always overpower all other actors and actions. Other factors can come into play which can challenge, resist, or offer reinterpretation, even where stigmatisation appears to be a highly fixed, territorialised process.

Stigma variation

Not only do stigmas have lineage in the past, but they also develop differentially over time, in relation to temporality, location, and sociocultural contexts. For example, initially, little was known about who was likely to get COVID-19 (and, thus, COVID-19 stigma). However, in the face of both new information and existing prejudices, the identification of 'others' occurred, usually along already established lineages of disadvantage. Indeed, those who are old, disabled, homeless, and/or from minoritised ethnic groups, those with pre-existing conditions or mental health problems, and those medically classified as 'overweight' or 'obese', are all more likely to have COVID-19 severely or die.

Farrimond (2021) identifies the double-edged sword of being identified in a group 'at-risk' in an epidemic. First, at-risk groups are often already disadvantaged and stigmatised; this is not surprising as most epidemics pattern along existing 'fault lines' in society, and COVID-19 is no exception (Roelen et al, 2020). Secondly, although being designated as an at-risk group allows for protection and prevention of transmission, it also risks identifying that whole group as a risk to the social body (Crawford, 1994). For this reason, I (HF) have argued that it is 'risky' for at-risk groups to be identified, both in terms of their social status and even their physical health (Farrimond, 2021).

The need to identify who is 'risky' is more pressing when considering COVID-19 compared to long COVID. Long COVID is not transmissible; it stops with the person who has it. Nevertheless, we see again signs of shame and blame towards those who have long COVID travelling down existing fault lines in society. Take, for example, a widely viewed meta-analysis of what factors make long COVID more likely, published in 2023 in the *Journal of the American Medical Association* (Tsampasian et al, 2023). This review of 41 studies found that the top factors that contributed to long COVID risk were not changeable – namely age (being over 40), sex (being female), and being in hospital for co-morbidities or severe COVID-19. Nevertheless, media articles, such as one in *The Washington Times*, published a summary of this paper with the emphasis on the 'lifestyle' risks such as smoking and higher BMI (body mass index)/obesity for long COVID, even though these risk factors were less prominent in the study (Salai, 2023).

The potential for individualising people's ill-health to cause shame and blame has been extensively detailed in medical sociology (Petersen and Lupton, 1996). Both smoking and being overweight are intensely stigmatised in the Global North (Farrimond and Joffe, 2006; Throsby, 2007), but are also known to be difficult to modify. It is interesting that the newspaper article did not lead with the one more easily modifiable preventive behaviour detailed in the paper, which was to have two or more vaccinations. Rather, the focus was on 'unhealthy life choices', with the underlying (othering) message being that healthy people will not get this, and those that do must deserve it. As such, it could be understood as a form of the weaponisation of stigma in action (Scambler, 2018).

The study also leads us to think about the role of gender in long COVID stigma. Long COVID stigma is not fully gendered in that both men and women can get long COVID. Several prominent sportsmen and sportswomen have provided accounts of being debilitated (Guardian Sport, 2022). However, overall, the risk for women may be as much as three-fold higher than for men (Bai et al, 2022). What are the consequences for long COVID stigma? Middle-aged/older women already have a long history of being made invisible within healthcare systems as well as more widely in society (Pérez, 2019). It is unlikely that those with long COVID will buck this trend. Long COVID is also associated with being in a lower socioeconomic group or having prior financial difficulties (Durstenfeld et al, 2023), which are then compounded by long COVID itself. Long COVID is, thus, the product of a cluster of existing stigmas, the effect of which is to amplify any resultant stigma.

Variation is, of course, related to adaptability to an environment. With respect to variation in stigmatisation, its sociocultural environment is highly fluid and multiple, which raises the issue of how we might best grasp variation. One way of doing this is by thinking of variation as a recruitment of the stigmatisation under investigation – in this case, long COVID – to other existing stigmatisations. That is, long COVID can be linked – that is, territorialised – through its association with groups already subject to stigmatisation (such as women and those who supposedly indulge in 'unhealthy lifestyle choices'). These can be further situated within broader assemblages that, for example, attribute the problems faced by a health service to 'unwarranted demand' as opposed to governmental underfunding. Still, it is important that we remain sensitised to potential de-territorialisations, for example, accounts of sportspeople who suffer long COVID.

Stigma strength

Stigma strength does not, as a term, say anything about any given incidence of stigma. Rather, it is used as a term to explain larger macro-waves of stigma, which amplify and decrease. Such stigma 'can amplify at particular cultural moments, but also weaken, producing less virulent strains, either deliberately through anti-stigma public health interventions or through broader cultural processes' (Farrimond, 2021, 181). If up to 95 per cent of people with long COVID experience stigma (Pantelic et al, 2022), we are surely in that cultural moment of stigma amplification. Why is this?

One way of understanding stigma strength is in terms of the number and range of connections that are aligned within an assemblage. The more in number and diversity, then the more potent and resonant a stigma is. Sometimes, this growth is deliberately pursued as part of an ideological deployment of stigma. We have already suggested an instance of this in the alignment – territorialisation – of long COVID, namely 'unhealthy lifestyle choices' and an 'unwarranted demand' on a health service. At other times, such territorialisation is harder to define.

Let us consider the symbolic social meaning of long COVID at this moment in time. Wars against disease are traumatic. Debates over their danger, meaning, and significance continue afterward. Some claim that the COVID-19 pandemic is not over. Booster vaccines are still in use. However, outward signs of engagement (for example, mass wearing of masks) are low. COVID-19 is not the core topic of social conversation that it was. For many, having COVID-19 has been downgraded to a mention and some sympathy, like having flu. What is discussed more avidly is the trauma the pandemic has caused, for example, whether the mental health of young people has declined and whether there is a general trauma-induced malaise settling over the population. Many people seem to simply want to forget, to move on. What, then, of those who have long COVID who may not be able to move on?

De Waal (2021) has written about the issue of collective memory in relation to epidemics in history. Epidemics which conform to the 'war metaphor' narrative, where we wage war against a disease but science/medicine triumphs (for example, as with cholera), are remembered as heroic episodes of human accomplishment. Others, such as the Spanish Flu (influenza) pandemic of 1916–1918, follow a different story. De Waal characterises the influenza pandemic as 'The Joker' which tricked the weakened population that had survived the Great (First World) War. Spanish Flu killed between 60 and 100 million, and then left the world stage, with no obvious medical victory. De Waal argues that, in terms of collective memory, the Great War flu story is particularly quietly told. Indeed, prior to the COVID-19 pandemic, many knew little or nothing about it.

De Waal suggests various reasons for this, such as collective shock, the desire to move on to the optimistic Roaring Twenties (or, rather, the Roaring Twenties were an attempt at collective forgetting), or the fact that it represents a failure of science rather than a victory. Post-pandemics, we might argue, is a war waged between those who want to forget and those who do not (or cannot). In the context of the removal of the social and regulatory aspects of COVID-19 control, long COVID survivors are an emotionally potent reminder of the pandemic that many would rather forget. People with long COVID talk about being 'ghosted', the deliberate hiding away, or invalidation, of their experience. Tyler (2020) reminds us of the materiality of stigma; the origins of the word come from the marking of slaves' bodies. Those with long COVID embody the traumatic recent past, the ongoing (hidden) present, and future vulnerabilities – in other words, scary and unpleasant things that people want to forget or ignore.

Furthermore, in light of government failures, it has become expedient to diminish the COVID-19 pandemic as a live political topic. One upshot is that paying due attention to long COVID formally within healthcare systems becomes less appealing to those in power, economically as well as politically. Here, the amplification of stigma is often diffusely symbolic, emotional, and embodied. Heterogeneous elements that straddle, for instance, scientific ambiguities, widespread affective unease, and vague collective memorialisation, coalesce to give further weight to, and amplify, long COVID stigmatisation. Here, the assemblage of long COVID topologically accumulates associations that are distant in time and space yet enhance its resonance. Put simply, more and more diffuse references to long COVID combine to give it additional social and political significance.

Of course, as we have stressed throughout, de-amplification is also possible. Such cumulations of connections and, thus, growth of stigma can be actively resisted, not least by problematising various constitutive connections. Destigmatisation does not just appear; it emerges in relation to existing stigma. Actors take up their positions in relation to something, not nothing. As they are more successful, and as cultural shifts emerge, counter-positions also emerge or are re-engaged. Examples of this would include: academics and clinicians writing and campaigning about long COVID (Callard and Perego, 2021); online support sites; advocacy groups, such as Long COVID Work or Long COVID International; and guidance from professional bodies on long COVID policies in the workplace. Equally, however, existing hierarchies and organisational actors can then swing into position to maintain the status quo (for example, problems accessing COVID-19 specialists; conflating of COVID-19 with other contested illnesses like ME). While activists can promote counter-positions that challenge stigmatising discourses, it is perhaps the more deep-seated connections that embed long COVID stigma among a broad range of social and cultural elements that offer the most resistance to destigmatising change.

Conclusion

This chapter has traced several of the empirical complexities associated with long COVID stigmatisation. Long COVID has served as a case study through which to explore 'stigma mutation' theory (Farrimond, 2021). As we have noted, 'stigma mutation' conceptualises the emergence and change over time of stigma in terms of three dimensions: 'lineage', 'variation', and 'strength'. The case of long COVID has also enabled us to expand on 'stigma mutation' theoretically. We argue that these three dimensions need to be treated as interconnected within what we call an 'assemblage'. The case of long COVID stigmatisation suggests a picture of stigmatisation as a shifting array of interrelations, that is, an 'assemblage' which is simultaneously territorialised (predictable) and de-territorialised (unpredictable).

In brief, to the extent that long COVID stigma has intensified as problematic, it has inspired us to offer a broader tentative framework for understanding stigma processes. Culturally and theoretically, we have attempted to read both long COVID and stigma processes in terms of an 'assemblage' of often heterogeneous elements, simultaneously stigmatising and destigmatising, territorialising and de-territorialising. Within this assemblage framework, we can attune our analysis not only to the intensity of long COVID stigma at this cultural moment, and the collective desire to forget or 'move on', but also to the possibilities that this may change in complex and not always predictable ways. Our hope is that this assemblage perspective will allow future processes of stigmatisation (and destigmatisation) to be fruitfully analysed.

Could things be different?

- Stigmas are not fixed or permanent. They can change, or 'mutate', over time. Understanding stigma processes helps us to identify where we can challenge and change stigma for the future.
- Stigmas also vary across different locations and environments in terms of sociocultural meanings, practices, and material factors (as part of stigma 'assemblages'). It is important, if we want to counter stigma, to pay attention to local variations.
- Stigmatisation can be both predictable and unpredictable. Stigma is predictable as it often intensifies around already disadvantaged groups. Knowing about the predictability of stigma can motivate us to ensure existing marginalised groups are not further stigmatised. Unpredictability can occur when new knowledge, actors, or events disrupt stigma processes. Paying attention to the unpredictability of stigma gives hope that it can be disrupted.

References

Ansell Pearson, K. (1999) *Germinal Life: The Difference and Repetition of Deleuze*, London: Routledge.

Bagcchi, S. (2020) 'Stigma during the COVID-19 pandemic', *The Lancet Infectious Diseases*, 20(7): 782.

Bai, F., Tomasoni, D., Falcinella, C., Barbanotti, D., Castoldi, R., Mulè, G. et al (2022) 'Female gender is associated with long COVID syndrome: A prospective cohort study', *Clinical Microbiology and Infection*, 28(4): 611.e9–16.

Ballering, A., Hartman, T.O. and Rosmalen, J. (2021) 'Long COVID-19, persistent somatic symptoms and social stigmatisation', *Journal of Epidemiology and Community Health*, 75(6): 603–4.

Callard, F, and Perego, E. (2021) 'How and why patients made Long Covid', *Social Science and Medicine*, 268: 113426.

Carel, H. (2024) Personal communication with HF, 19 April.
Chaichana, U., Man, K.K.C., Chen, A., Wong, I.C.K., George, J, Wilson, P. and Wei, L. (2023) 'Definition of post–COVID-19 condition among published research studies', *JAMA Network Open*, 6(4): e235856.
Choi, S. (2021) "People look at me like I AM the virus': Fear, stigma, and discrimination during the COVID-19 pandemic', *Qualitative Social Work*, 20(1–2): 233–39.
Clarke, J. (1997) 'Capturing the customer? Consumerism and social welfare', *Self, Agency and Society*, 1(2): 55–73.
Cooper, F., Dolezal, L. and Rose, A. (2023) *COVID-19 and Shame: Political Emotions and Public Health in the UK*, London, New York, and Dublin: Bloomsbury Academic.
Crawford, R. (1994) 'The boundaries of the self and the unhealthy other: Reflections on health, culture and AIDS', *Social Science and Medicine*, 38(10): 1347–65.
Damant, R.W., Rourke, L., Cui, Y., Lam, G.Y., Smith, M.P., Fuhr, D.P. et al (2023) 'Reliability and validity of the post COVID-19 condition stigma questionnaire: A prospective cohort study', *eClinicalMedicine*, 55: 101755.
Darling-Hammond, S., Michaels, E.K., Allen, A.M., Chae, D.H., Thomas, M.D., Nguyen, T.T. et al (2020) 'After "the China virus" went viral: Racially charged coronavirus coverage and trends in bias against Asian Americans', *Health Education and Behaviour*, 47(6): 870–79.
Davis, H.E., McCorkell, L., Vogel, J. M. and Topol, E.J. (2023) 'Long COVID: Major findings, mechanisms and recommendations', *Nature Reviews Microbiology*, 21(3): 133–46.
Deleuze, G., and Guattari, F. (1988) *A Thousand Plateaus: Capitalism and Schizophrenia*, London: Athlone Press.
De Waal, A. (2021) *New Pandemics, Old Politics: Two Hundred Years of War on Disease and its Alternatives*, Polity Press: Cambridge, UK.
Durstenfeld, M.S., Peluso, M.J., Peyser, N.D., Lin, F., Knight, S.J., Djibo, A. et al (2023) 'Factors associated with long COVID symptoms in an online cohort study', *Open Forum Infectious Diseases*,10(2): ofad047.
Farrimond, H. (2021) 'Stigma mutation: Tracking lineage, variation and strength in emerging COVID-19 stigma', *Sociological Research Online*, 28(1): 171–88.
Farrimond, H. and Joffe, H. (2006) 'Pollution, peril and poverty: A British study of the stigmatization of smokers', *Journal of Community and Applied Social Psychology*, 16(6): 481–91.
Froelich, L., Hattesohl, D.B., Cotler, J., Jason, L.A., Scheibenbogen, C. and Behrends, U. (2022) 'Causal attributions and perceived stigma for myalgic encephalomyelitis/chronic fatigue syndrome', *Journal of Health Psychology*, 27(10): 2290–2304.

Garner, P. (2021) 'Paul Garner: On his recovery from long Covid', *The BMJ Opinion*, [online] 25 January, Available from: https://blogs.bmj.com/bmj/2021/01/25/paul-garner-on-his-recovery-from-long-covid/ [Accessed 28 January 2025].

Goffman, E. (1963) *Stigma: Notes on the Management of Spoiled Identity*, Englewood Cliffs, NJ: Prentice-Hall.

Guardian Sport (2022) 'NHL's Brandon Sutter says long Covid has sidelined him for entire season', *The Guardian*, [online] 27 April, Available from: https://www.theguardian.com/sport/2022/apr/27/brandon-sutter-long-covid-nhl-ice-hockey-vancouver-canucks [Accessed 28 January 2025].

Gui, L. (2021) 'Media framing of fighting COVID-19 in China', *Sociology of Health and Illness*, 43(4): 966–70.

Jackson, J.E. (2008) 'Stigma, liminality, and chronic pain: Mind–body borderlands', *American Ethnologist*, 32(3): 332–53.

Jones, E.E., Farina, A., Hastorf, A.H., Markus, H., Miller, D.T. and Scott, R.A. (1984) *Social Stigma: The Psychology of Marked Relationships*, New York: Freeman.

Latour, B. (2005) *Reassembling the Social: An Introduction to Actor-Network-Theory*, Oxford: Oxford University Press.

Latour, B. (2010) 'Steps toward the writing of a compositionist manifesto', *New Literary History*, 41: 471–90.

Lindsay, J. (2022) 'The stigma of Long Covid: Why people don't believe it's real', *Metro*, [online] 16 March, Available from: https://metro.co.uk/2022/03/16/the-stigma-of-long-covid-why-people-dont-believe-its-real-16217101/ [Accessed 28 January 2025].

Link, B.G., and Phelan, J.C. (2001) 'Conceptualizing stigma', *Annual Review of Sociology*, 27: 363–85.

MacPherson, K., Cooper, K., Harbour, J., Mahal, D., Miller, C. and Nairn, M. (2022) 'Experiences of living with long COVID and of accessing healthcare services: A qualitative systematic review', *BMJ Open*, 12(1): e050979.

Mathioudakis, A.G., Ananth, S. and Vestbo, J. (2021) 'Stigma: An unmet public health priority in COPD', *The Lancet: Respiratory Medicine*, 9(9): 955–6.

Michael, M. (2017) *Actor-Network Theory: Trials, Trails and Translations*, London: SAGE Publications.

Mol, A. (2002) *The Body Multiple: Ontology in Medical Practice*, Durham, NC: Duke University Press.

Morrison, C. (2023) 'A FIFTH of "long Covid" sufferers haven't returned to work a year later', *The Daily Mail*, [online] 24 January, Available from: https://www.dailymail.co.uk/health/article-11671041/A-FIFTH-long-Covid-sufferers-havent-returned-work-year-later.html [Accessed 28 January 2025].

Pantelic, M., and Alwan, N. (2021) 'The stigma is real for people living with long covid', *The BMJ Opinion*, [online] 25 March, Available from: https://blogs.bmj.com/bmj/2021/03/25/marija-pantelic-and-nisreen-alwan-the-stigma-is-real-for-people-living-with-long-covid/ [Accessed 15 March 2023].

Pantelic, M., Ziauddeen, N., Boyes, M., O'Hara, M.E., Hastie, C. and Alwan, N.A. (2022) 'Long Covid stigma: Estimating burden and validating scale in a UK-based sample' *PLOS ONE*, 17(11): e0277317.

Perego, E., Callard, F. and Stras, L., Melville-Jóhannesson, B., Pope, R. and Alwan, N.A. (2020) 'Why the patient-made term "Long Covid" is needed', *Wellcome Open Research*, 5: 224.

Pérez, C.C. (2019) *Invisible Women: Data Bias in a World Designed for Men*, London: Chatto & Windus.

Petersen, A., and Lupton, D. (1996) *The New Public Health: Health and Self in an Age of Risk*, Thousand Oaks, CA: Sage Publications Inc.

Roelen, K., Ackley, C., Boyce, P., Farina, N. and Ripoll, S. (2020) 'COVID-19 in LMICs: The need to place stigma front and centre to its response', *European Journal of Development Research*, 32(5): 1592–1612.

Salai, S. (2023) 'Study links "long COVID" to unhealthy life choices', *The Washington Times*, [online] 23 March, Available from: https://www.washingtontimes.com/news/2023/mar/23/study-links-long-covid-unhealthy-life-choices/ [Accessed 28 January 2025].

Scambler, G. (2018) 'Heaping blame on shame: "Weaponising stigma" for neoliberal times', *The Sociological Review*, 66(4): 766–82.

Spandler, H. and Allen, M. (2018) 'Contesting the psychiatric framing of ME/CFS', *Social Theory and Health*, 16(2): 127–41.

Strong, P. (1990) 'Epidemic psychology: A model', *Sociology of Health & Illness*, 12(3): 249–59.

The Lancet (2023) 'Long COVID: 3 years in', *The Lancet*, 401(10379): 795.

Throsby, K. (2007) '"How could you let yourself get like that?": Stories of the origins of obesity in accounts of weight loss surgery', *Social Science and Medicine*, 65(8): 1561–71.

Tsampasian, V., Elghazaly, H., Chattopadhyay, R. and Debski, N. (2023) 'Risk factors associated with post–COVID-19 condition: A systematic review and meta-analysis', *JAMA Internal Medicine*, 183(6): 566–80.

Tyler, I. (2020) *Stigma: The Machinery of Inequality*, London: Zed Books Ltd.

Tyler, I., and Slater, T. (2018) 'Rethinking the sociology of stigma', *The Sociological Review*, 66(4): 721–43.

World Health Organization (2022) 'Increasing recognition, research and rehabilitation for post COVID-19 condition (long COVID)', *World Health Organization*, [online], Available from: https://www.who.int/europe/activities/increasing-recognition-research-and-rehabilitation-for-post-covid-19-condition-long-covid [Accessed 28 January 2025].

9

Notes on a Spoiled Working Identity: Stigma, Illness, and Disability in the Contemporary (Western) Workplace

Jennifer Remnant

Introduction

This chapter focuses on the workplace stigmatisation of disabled workers and workers experiencing long-term ill-health. Despite the chapter title, which cites Goffman (1963), this chapter draws on Imogen Tyler's (2020) definition of stigma, positing stigmatisation as a form of oppression. Though there is extensive research and theorising that highlights the stigma related to being unemployed, whether disabled or not (Bambra, 2011; Karren and Sherman, 2012), far less work has focused on workplace enactments of stigma and their impact on disabled workers. A relatively recent proliferation of academic work relating to organisational equality, diversity, and inclusion (EDI) policies, strategies, and agendas implies an increased interest in the experiences of disadvantaged, oppressed, and marginalised people at work (Gould et al, 2022; Tompa et al, 2022), and a shared recognition that workplace policies, including those designed to promote equality, are broadly failing to meet the needs of these workers (Pilkington, 2020; Remnant et al, 2024).

This chapter extends critique of workplace human resource management (HRM) policies to argue that, in contemporary UK workplaces, the implementation of organisational HRM policies and practices *are* an enactment of stigma against disabled and ill workers. Disabled and ill workers deviate from the unobtainable and constructed standards of the ideal worker (Acker, 1990) and are required, instead, to meet the exacting standards of the 'sick role' (Parsons, 1951), which are similarly unobtainable. Thus, disabled workers and workers with long-term health conditions are trapped in a position where they are deemed unable to be adequately non-disabled/well enough to be worthwhile employees but are not ill enough to deserve changes in practice or improved accessibility.

There are two key practical elements of this stigmatisation. The first is the situating of disabled workers by policy as an issue of absence or poor performance rather than retention. The second is the additional labour required of these workers to either 'pass' as not-ill/disabled or repeatedly having to disclose their condition to negotiate access to workplace support – both of which, ironically, can inhibit performance. Disabled workers are stigmatised at work by the processes and assumptions central *to* work. Supportive management at work, by nature of the assumptions underpinning human resources (HR) policies, is conditional for disabled workers dependent on their proximity to the ideal worker or the sick role. It makes employment precarious and disadvantages disabled people, despite the often good intentions of managers.

I begin the chapter by exploring the relationship between morality and work in the UK and outlining the concept of the ideal worker. From here, I discuss contemporary understandings of deservingness in relation to Parsons' (1951) 'sick role' and apply those to the workplace. The chapter moves on to use empirical research data to detail how HR policies stigmatise disabled and long-term ill workers, before illustrating the additional labour required of already disadvantaged workers.

This chapter draws on the perspectives and experiences of multiple stakeholders regarding the management and support of disabled employees and those with long-term health conditions or symptoms. The chapter draws on published and unpublished data from a variety of projects that I have been involved with or led on, all of which are interview-based (Remnant, 2017, 2019, 2021; Sang, Calvard et al, 2021; Sang, Remnant et al, 2021; Remnant et al, 2022, 2024). Details of the studies/papers are provided in Table 9.1 as well as in the reference list. Participants include line managers, HR staff, occupational health staff, healthcare professionals, and employees experiencing long-term health conditions and/or impairment. This includes people with 'leaky bodies', namely, bodies that involuntarily excrete fluids including blood, sweat, faeces, and urine.

I use the descriptor 'disabled people' in this chapter, rather than the person-first language of 'people with disabilities'. This is in keeping with the social model of disability, which has political utility when discussing disability. The model focuses on ableist societal perspectives and norms and enables a political categorisation of disability, long-term ill-health, and long-term undiagnosed symptoms. It allows us to analyse the experiences of everyone who is disadvantaged by ableism and ableist practices, whether

Table 9.1: Studies referenced

Study focus/ title	Principle investigator	Publications
Who gets what? Negotiating work and welfare after a cancer diagnosis	Jen Remnant	Remnant, J. (2017) *Who Gets What? Negotiating Work and Welfare after a Cancer Diagnosis.* Unpublished PhD Thesis: Newcastle University. Remnant, J. (2019) 'Getting what you deserve: How notions of deservingness feature in the experiences of employees with cancer', *Social Science and Medicine*, 237(September): 112447. Remnant, J. (2021) 'Managing cancer in contemporary workforces: How employees with cancer and line managers negotiate post-diagnosis support in the workplace', *Employee Relations*, 44(1): 229–43.
Disability inclusive science careers	Kate Sang	Remnant, J. Sang, K., Calvard, T., Richards, J. and Babajide, O. (2024) 'Exclusionary logics: Constructing disability and disadvantaging disabled academics in the neoliberal university', *Sociology*, 58(1): 23–44.
Academics with gynaecological health conditions	Kate Sang	Sang, K., Remnant, J., Calvard, T. and Myhill, K. (2021) 'Blood work: Managing menstruation, menopause and gynaecological health conditions in the workplace', *International Journal of Environmental Research and Public Health*, 18(4): 1951.
Leaky bodies	Jen Remnant	Remnant, J. Sang, K., Myhill, K., Calvard, T., Chowdhry, S. and Richards, J. (2022) 'Working it out: Will the improved management of leaky bodies in the workplace create a dialogue between medical sociology and disability studies?', *Sociology of Health and Illness*, 45(6): 1276–99.
Disabled Academics	Kate Sang	Sang, K., Calvard, T. and Remnant, J. (2021) 'Disability and academic careers: Using the social model to reveal the role of human resource management practices in creating disability, *Work, Employment and Society*, 36(4): 722–40.

they are legally, medically, or self-defined as disabled or do not identify with disability at all. The social model situates disability in terms of the verb 'disable'. We are disabled by ableism. As such, in this chapter, stigmatisation is considered a disabling practice with social and material implications for disabled and ill workers.

The ideal worker and the sick role

The concept of the 'ideal worker' refers to a set of characteristics and expectations associated with an idealised employee in the workplace (Acker,

1990; Reid, 2015). The ideal worker possesses traits such as unwavering commitment and dedication to their job, a strong work ethic, long hours of availability, and a willingness (and ability) to prioritise work over other life responsibilities, including caring roles and their personal wellbeing (Reid, 2015; Sang et al, 2015). These values are desirable to employers. When these traits are embraced by a worker, there is evidence that they are rewarded, particularly for people in white-collar professions or managerial roles, with progression, benefits, and bonuses (Bailyn, 2016). The ideal worker is the embodiment of neoliberalism: increased performance to ensure maximum profitability (Telford and Briggs, 2022) and an extreme manifestation of the broader relationship in Western societies of work to morality.

In the Western context, the worthiness of someone's citizenship is tied up with their employment and work status (Bambra, 2011). When asked 'what do you do?', we recognise that we are being asked our occupation – what we do for money, not what we do for leisure. There is wide agreement among sociologists exploring stigma, work, and welfare that the primary requirement made of the citizen in the Global North is to contribute to society by means of paid work (Ekerdt, 1986; Bambra, 2011; Patrick, 2012; Frayne, 2015). It is the method by which participants in a society become full citizens, evidencing productivity and contribution (Handler, 2003; Larkin, 2011; Tyler, 2020). There are few conditions under which a person is deemed morally deserving of respite from work, and fewer still in public opinion, to receive State welfare.

Van Oorschot and Roosma (2017) have researched public perceptions of deservingness and have identified five criteria that an individual must meet to be deemed to be deserving of welfare payments. These criteria are control, attitude, reciprocity, identity, and need, coined the CARIN criteria for deservingness. Control means that the deserving individual is not in control of their situation, or responsible for their misfortune. Attitude is the expectation that those deemed deserving should be suitably grateful for the support they receive. Reciprocity as a criterion reflects the perceived responsibility of benefit claimants to earn the support they receive: the more reciprocation, the more deserving. Identity refers to someone being part of society, and not 'other'. The last criterion relates to need: the greater an individual's need, the more deserving they are of State welfare (Van Oorschot, 2000).

The CARIN criteria reflect, to some extent, the exchange fundamental to some medical sociological theorising around ill-health. Talcott Parsons (1951) outlined the nature of the criteria for acceptable deviance from ordinary duties (identified here as paid employment) in his theorising of the 'sick role'. According to the sick role model, being ill must include a reciprocal exchange of duties for entitlements (Parsons, 1951). The duties of an ill person are to seek out and comply with competent help in the form of medical expertise, and to make all attempts to get better (Varul, 2010). The corresponding entitlements of the sick role for people experiencing ill health are to not be blamed for their illness and temporary exemption from their normal duties while they recover. Varul (2010, 83) explains that the 'classical sick role requires patients to dedicate all their efforts and time to prepare for normality after the sick role'.

Not only does this replicate the CARIN criteria, but it also reflects how illness is managed and conceptualised in relation to work. Our working systems have been designed for workers to take sick leave when ill, get better, and then return to work. Illness, within this model, is temporally bounded, time limited, and temporary. Despite the age of Parsons' theorising, it is (unintentionally) supported in more contemporary health literature, which so often focuses on a return to work as a significant milestone for recovery for people experiencing ill-health (Kennedy et al, 2007; Wells et al, 2013).

Charmaz (2000) notes that, in contrast with the assumptions of the sick role, people with chronic (long-term) conditions do not recover. Parsons, however, refuted that the sick role inadequately explained long-term conditions in a later publication (Parsons, 1975). Defence of the sick role has included the suggestion that people with long-term conditions might be subject to different expectations from their acutely ill peers (Kassebaum and Baumann, 1965), or that a return to normal duties could result from the successful management of their condition (Parsons, 1975). However, this presumes an unchanging, static condition rather than the long-term social process of many conditions that can include degeneration and/or fluctuation (Nettleton, 2006) or the experiences of disabled people who are not ill.

The sick role links illness to absence from work, which mirrors a wider societal conceptualisation of disability as being in opposition to the completion of paid work. Notably few historic depictions of work and employment include acknowledgement of disability (UK National Archives, n.d.), despite health conditions and impairments having always been a feature of human diversity. Historically, poor and working-class disabled and ill people (and current workers with no recourse to social welfare funds) must have worked to survive, whether that work was subsistence-based or waged labour. Despite this, there is an enduring assumption in policy and practice in the UK that disability and ill-health are defined by the inability to complete paid work. It is in response to this assumption, and the subsequent exclusion of disabled people from economic participation (the disability employment gap), that disabled scholars and activists developed disability studies and the social model of disability (Shakespeare, 2006).

Despite considerable critique of the sick role with its limited explanatory potential for long-term conditions, its enduring presence and common usage as a model for illness should not be underestimated. The sick role, and the functionalist framework in which it resides, continues to complement the organisation of work and employment in the UK (Brown and Rawlinson, 1977; Bellaby, 1990), as it is 'basically economic' (Gerhardt, 1979, 231). The sick role reflects the preferences of employers, and of the State, to assume a workforce of ideal workers and have those unable to work because of sickness back to work as soon as possible (Bellaby, 1990). The model is a single element of a 'much larger set of mechanics embedded in the social system: a "window" effectively, on a broader set of motivational balances' (Williams, 2005, 130).

Significantly, for a discussion of stigma, a central issue with Parsons' sick role thesis is that it does not problematise the power structures it describes (Johnson, 1972) and assumes passivity rather than agency within the ill and/ or disabled population (Radley, 1994). This raises a complexity in how stigma manifests within this model. Though we can recognise how being disabled, being ill, or being 'leaky' can be stigmatised, the purpose of the sick role is to legitimise being ill through specific obligations and is not necessarily a stigmatised position. Drawing on interview data from a selection of research projects, the rest of this chapter explores when, why, and how some disabled or ill people move out of the legitimised sick role and into a stigmatised position in the workplace or never fulfil the sick role at all.

Appropriate absence or poor performance

There is an enduring reluctance to recruit, retain, or promote disabled people in all work sectors and work types (Bonaccio et al, 2020). Unsurprisingly, a result of this has been a sustained gap between the proportion of disabled people of working age who are in paid work, and the proportion of non-disabled people in paid work, referred to as the disability employment gap (Sainsbury, 2018). When able to access paid work, disabled people are likely to be underemployed, that is, employed below their ability/qualification level, and/or be in part-time or fixed term rather than full-time work (Rozali et al, 2017) due to the negative views that recruiters and managers hold about disabled workers' potential performance.

A key contributor to these views is the policy framework used in Western workplaces. As described earlier, work and disability have been constructed in opposition to each other in the Western legislative context, and this has been replicated within employing organisations. There is a social construction of disability in UK workplaces, in that useful information regarding the support and management of disabled people is located in absence and capability policies – rather than EDI policies – which only contain rhetoric and information on minimum legal practice (Remnant et al, 2024). This means that when a disabled or long-term ill worker discloses a condition, diagnosis, or symptom to their manager, the manager is directed toward policies that define disability as a problem.

The idea that ill-health or disability is a binary experience of ill-and-absent or recovered-and-at-work has been implicit and explicit in managerial testimony. Employers recognise and describe the unacceptable middle option of being off work when 'better'. The following quote is from an occupational health manager working in the public sector describing when and how she encourages employees with cancer to return to work: 'I can actually say to somebody who's off … I think it's time you went back to work, you know, you're getting to the point now where you need to be back at work because you-, there's only so much Jeremy Kyle any one person can watch' (Remnant, 2017, 126). This quote is telling in terms of what the manager assumes employees do when absent, as it corresponds with problematic stereotypes relating to worklessness and how people out of work are stigmatised (Gavin, 2021). This participant also provided an account of supporting two employees with similar long-term health conditions. She explained how one of the employees was admirable, because he did everything in his power to come back to work as soon as possible, whereas the other took his full sick leave entitlement. Most offensively, to her, he was seen to be 'living his life' while on sick leave – visiting a pub, no less. She suggested that the employee being at the pub was evidence that he was well enough to work but choosing not to. She explained that when he returned to work, his colleagues made his life 'miserable' on this basis and he left the job not long after. He was stigmatised, with material effect, not because he was ill, but because he was not ill *enough* to be absent and, as such, did not fulfil the perceived obligations of an ill employee.

The data illustrate how disabled and ill workers are offered a binary option of the ideal worker or the sick worker – neither of which reflect the fluctuating and long-term symptoms that represent contemporary experiences of ill-health and/or disability. Good employees are either at work and evidencing a strong work ethic and good performance, or are unwell and perhaps absent, though demonstrating a strong desire to return to work.

Disability and/or long-term ill-health are also managed via capability or performance policies (sometimes also related to absence). Many workplace policies are explicit that managers are required to identify whether an employee's reduced performance is for a legitimate reason, which would include *genuine* ill-health or disability. It is less clear how managers are expected to make this distinction between genuine and legitimate illness and disingenuous claims of ill-health. Many organisations have the option to access occupational health expertise but are not required to follow the guidance provided. This absence of clear direction exposes employee support to managerial discretion, and though this could have potential benefits for disabled employees, it often appears informed by problematic assumptions surrounding disability, illness, and capability, and incorrect interpretations of the Equality Act (2010): 'The university, quite rightly actually, provides zero support unless you're diagnosed' (Research Leader, in Remnant et al, 2024, 37). This participant implies that employees can only access support from the employer relating to their illness or impairment if they have a diagnosis. This is directly at odds with the Equality Act (2010), which only states that an individual must have experienced or expect to experience symptoms for over twelve months, not that they must have a clinical diagnosis. This is important as many individuals will experience symptoms for years before (and if) they are diagnosed, especially with gynaecological (Endometriosis UK, 2023) or neurodiverse conditions (British Medical Association, 2019).

When not absent from work, disabled employees and employees with long-term health conditions describe having their performance queried by managers and colleagues when they disclose impairment effects (Remnant et al, 2024). Across all the projects I have been involved with, there has been the shared worry among managers about what they should or should not say to an employee disclosing ill-health, symptoms, or a condition. Managers have frequently described using HR colleagues to outsource responsibility for difficult conversations about performance, particularly if relating to a performance procedure. These conversations are difficult because they are avoided in the first instance, meaning that the issues experienced by disabled and ill individuals at work are often only identified when a crisis point is reached.

Even when not engaged in a performance procedure involving HR, discomfort around open conversations with employees can translate into an obstacle to progression. When disability is disclosed, managers no longer explore employee progression and accomplishments, instead informing employees that they are doing well for 'coping' with their conditions or symptoms (Sang, Calvard et al, 2021; Sang, Remnant et al, 2021) or avoiding the topic of their health completely. Here, the practice of stigmatisation is slower and more subtle than the stigmatisation attached to inappropriate absence. Instead of immediate shaming, disabled people and those with long-term health conditions can experience a plateauing of their career, the slow-burn humiliation of being left behind by their contemporaries, with no obvious recourse to contestation and unspoken implications of reduced performance.

Data from line managers and HR professionals echo the experiences of disabled workers. In interviews about supporting disabled employees or those with long-term health conditions, decision makers are often unable to explain how they would apply EDI policy content to support employees with promotion and/or progression. The following quote is from a senior member of HR staff working for a higher education employer and illustrates the difficulties in the logistics of acknowledging disability or long-term ill-health as part of the promotions procedure: 'We are looking at reviewing our academic promotions policy and specifically putting something in there that says, you know, allowances should be made for breaks in service and things like that. But practically, how that would work, I don't know' (Remnant et al, 2024, 35). The participant reflects on absence as the key issue disabled or long-term ill employees might experience and, even then, does not know how she and her team would instrumentalise support for said employees in a revised organisational policy. It would seem practicable to make allowances for breaks in service, given that these result from life experiences other than ill-health, including parental or care-related leave. There is an implied exceptionalism to disability here, that separates it from other absences from work – an unspoken stigmatisation based on assumptions about future performance that are not made about other colleagues who experience absence from work. Additionally, throughout the interview, this participant only spoke about absence, as if that would be the only difference between a worker with a long-term health condition and one without. She did not reflect on the potential to alter working practices or role expectations to accommodate the diversity inherent in disability and ill-health.

There is a clear problem with how we construct disability and/or illness in the workplace as an issue either of absence – which is policed as to whether it is appropriate – or (diminished) performance. If formalised as part of a performance procedure, line managers are expected to make decisions based on whether they believe their employee to be *genuinely* ill/disabled, despite infrequently being qualified to do so. If not formalised through a performance procedure, unspoken assumptions regarding employee capability inform decisions that often inhibit disabled colleagues or those with long-term health conditions from progressing and developing in the workplace. With these inadequate and inhibitive policy frameworks in place, it is necessary to reflect on why disabled or ill employees disclose their conditions, and what the implications of non-disclosure are.

Disclosure: masking or negotiating accommodations

From the previous sections, it is possible to speculate as to the reasons an employee might not disclose a health condition, ongoing symptoms, or disability to their manager. We have seen examples of mistreatment and mismanagement, even where the intention is good, and have seen how workplace policies with supportive aims are central to the workplace stigmatisation of disabled and long-term ill workers. However, that same policy context requires disclosure because it should enable the provision of lawful practice by employers (Grunfeld et al, 2013), placing individual workers in a catch-22. In this section, I explore the additional labour required of employees with long-term conditions to navigate disclosure.

Disclosure is complicated. An employee with cancer is likely to have disclosed their diagnosis and taken sick leave to access their treatment. In the years after they have returned to work, they might experience any number of cancer (treatment) related health issues, including anxiety, cognitive dysfunction, reduced mobility, pain, and/or fatigue. It becomes difficult at this point to pinpoint exactly what disclosure would be, unless the individual was well versed in their employee rights, and many are not informed or are unable to advocate for themselves while also managing their symptoms (Remnant, 2017). Certainly, there is a growing body of evidence that employees experiencing ill-health receive less support over time (Bramwell et al, 2016; Remnant, 2021) – and that there is an appropriate amount of time to 'get over' illness, *even* if it is cancer (Remnant, 2022). Alternatively, if an individual is at the beginning of their ill-health, disability, or diagnostic journey, it could well be that they feel as though they have nothing to disclose, or that the specific symptom they might disclose feels too stigmatised or embarrassing to bring up in the first instance.

For example, in research led by Kate Sang (Remnant et al, 2022, 1290), an academic employee described how she sought to hide her symptoms in the workplace: 'I don't walk between the students ... I'm scared my menstruation blood and scent is too strong.' For other employees, avoiding disclosure meant fully withdrawing from their work, often without the management of their health condition or subsequent stigmatised identity being shared as a causal factor. Participants were able to identify that disclosure actually enables the enactment of stigmatisation in the workplace. Though criticised for not engaging in the wider power relations implied by this, Goffman (1963) did identify the various ways that individuals who might be stigmatised attempt to manage their identity. Passing, covering, and withdrawing – all discussed by Goffman – align with the data presented. This included people medicating or working longer hours to make up for perceived disability-caused shortfalls. People experiencing fatigue, a symptom of numerous health conditions and impairments, would downplay and cover their feelings of fatigue by taking naps between meetings when working from home, or reducing their involvement in other leisure activities or hobbies.

This returns us to the problematic neoliberal construct of the ideal worker. Participants were aware that to disclose their health condition was to expose the distance between their reality and the impossible aspirations of the ideal worker (Sang et al, 2015). They were able to explain how non-disclosure was necessary to fulfil the requirements of their role, especially if their conditions were ongoing. The following quote comes from a participant with a long-term gynaecological health condition, where she discusses how the disclosure of her symptoms would undermine her professional credibility and make her problematic:

> This is so kind of anti-feminism, I wouldn't want to be problematic or it's something for me to manage and I don't agree with this at all,

but this is kind of how I approach it, it's something for me to manage and not kind of have to enforce that on anyone else. And yeah, so I suppose it's more about my professional credibility perhaps. (Remnant et al, 2022, 1290)

As with data from managers and HR professionals, this employee places being symptomatic at odds with being a good employee. It reinforces the binary position that employees should either be unwell and absent, or present and 'ideal'. It also raises the question of how employees who cannot 'pass' as not-disabled, not-symptomatic, or not-ill manage to navigate the workplace.

If not passing or withdrawing, stigmatised workers must identify and share their protected characteristic, ongoing symptoms, or (potential) diagnosis with their employer. As discussed previously, in the short-term, there is evidence that managers provide lots of support to employees experiencing ill-health, but that this diminishes over time (Bramwell, 2016). As support dwindles, or the specific access needs of a worker are forgotten or ignored, disclosure ceases to be a one-off conversation but instead evolves into an ongoing interaction between employees and employers. Rather than limitations related to their symptoms or impairment effect, disabled workers instead become limited by having to engage in the work of multiple disclosures to get adequate workplace support or accommodations. In the Equality Act (2010), these accommodations are referred to as 'reasonable adjustments'. Disabled people have long described the provision of workplace support as based on the goodwill of managers (Foster, 2007) rather than the enactment of their legal entitlements based on their membership of a group disadvantaged by an ableist society.

Disabled workers find themselves actively discredited in the workplace or have their concerns about meeting their targets belittled by their managers. One participant, working in a higher education institution, offered an illustrative account of this issue. She explained that she could not teach in a particular lecture hall due to her impairment. She confirmed this again with a new manager when she saw that she had been put down to work in that lecture hall the following semester. She described her manager's response: 'The reply I got from the new person was, "yes, I heard you don't like teaching in there. I'll see what I can do", and I thought, you know, that's not okay. It's not a preference' (Sang et al, 2022, 734). Ultimately, the employee reported that their management made them feel 'insubordinate' for requesting an accommodation, but also implies a disbelief about employee claims of ill-health or impairment. Disabled employees, including those with gynaecological health conditions, have explained how they were concerned that their managers thought they were complaining, when they should simply continue as they are.

In many cases, this has extended to being subject to resentment for getting support that other employees do not receive. Worse still, this included additional resentment on the basis that the individual was accessing this additional support but did not deserve it. Disclosure, of course, is further complicated by confidentiality, managerial changes, and staff turnover (Gignac et al, 2021). This concept of accessing support disingenuously or inappropriately allocates employees to a space that fails to meet either the exacting requirements of being an ideal worker or the obligations of the deserving sick role.

Once in this liminal space, isolated and stigmatised by both HR policies and managerial practice, employees are redirected from progression and development. Participants often discussed how, instead of exploring how their skills and knowledge could be retained appropriately, the reasonable adjustments they were offered were instead to reduce their hours or they were invited to discuss ways in which they could leave work, categorising them in opposition to the ideal full-time, productive, promotable, non-disabled workers. This was particularly so for employees with hidden impairments, gynaecological health issues or symptoms, and people who had recovered from acute episodes of ill-health and were experiencing longer-term, fluctuating symptoms.

Conclusion

This chapter illustrates how the workplace stigmatisation of disabled workers and workers experiencing long-term ill-health is enacted through workplace processes, including those that are (ostensibly) designed to support diversity in the workplace. The chapter has extended understandings of stigmatisation to critique workplace HRM policies, arguing that in contemporary UK workplaces, the implementation of organisational HRM policies and practices are an enactment of stigma against disabled and ill workers. Disabled and ill workers, representing a deviation from the unobtainable and constructed standards of the neoliberal ideal worker (Acker, 1990), are also unable to meet the exacting standards of the sick role (Parsons, 1951). This traps workers in a position where they are deemed unable to be adequately non-disabled/well enough to be worthwhile employees but are not ill or deserving enough to be absent. They enter a precarious space where difficult decisions must be made regarding disclosure (if they have a hidden impairment). To not disclose requires passing as a non-ill, non-symptomatic, or non-disabled worker, but leaves employees vulnerable to crises where exposure is forced, whereas disclosure is necessary to enable workplace support, but instead enables stigmatising practices. Workplace support becomes conditional for disabled workers dependent on their proximity to the ideal worker or the sick role. The unruly bodies of disabled or ill workers challenge the social organisation of the workplace, built as it is around unobtainable ideals – exaggerated by the rise in neoliberalism and associated competition and managerialism.

Could things be different?

Policy and legislative initiatives have been evidenced to be ineffective improving the experiences of disabled workers, and due to broader societal stigma, disabled people are limited in their opportunities to enact change in the workplace. As such, it is employers who are best placed to minimise the disability employment gap and reduce the stigmatised practices experienced by disabled workers, by:

- Focusing on skill retention: Employers can develop organisational strategies aiming to minimise turnover related to ill-health by focusing on skillsets they need to retain and recognising employees' organisational knowledge and experience. This would require employers to reflect on the investment of time and resource by employees into the organisation, and vice versa, to identify the ongoing value of that investment in the instance of employee illness and/or impairment. In practical terms, this can include discussing employee knowledge and experience in performance reviews and managerial check-in conversations.
- Acknowledging the value of diverse experiences: There is evidence that the representation of diverse experiences in a workforce can positively inform performance. Disabled workers and workers experiencing long term ill-health can draw on their previous experience of being an undiagnosed/non-symptomatic/non-disabled worker *and* their new experiences of being diagnosed/symptomatic/disabled. This learning will have value that can be operationalised to develop managerial practices.
- Developing new human resource practices, such as job crafting: This is an effective strategy to overcome the inaccessibility of the labour market by formally recognising the flexibility of task allocation within working roles. It is a common informal practice among working teams to distribute tasks depending on the strengths, limitations, and preferences of specific workers. It is possible to extend this into a formal practice to support all employees to perform at their best.
- Using accurate language and providing appropriate resources: Many Scottish employers make menstruation products available to their employees and include a supply in toilets labelled for men. This represents a simple acknowledgement that some workers menstruate, and it is more accurate to use the terminology of menstruation rather than 'feminine hygiene' or 'sanitary products'. A further improvement would be to provide incontinence products in employee toilets.

Within the academic and research community, we could also reframe how we consider disability and ill-health in relation to work:

- We need to conduct more research that does not position a 'return-to-work' as an outcome in and of itself. Along with the return to work, we need to explore the experience of those returns, whether employees are retained, and whether they progress. We need to reflect on what inhibits and/or enables progression or improved wellbeing for disabled and/or long-term ill workers.
- There needs to be a recognition in management literature that not all work is good. It is important that we clarify that *good* work is associated with better health outcomes, not *any* work.
- Academic work often shies away from describing the specifics of ill-health. By using palatable and euphemistic language, we undermine the material experiences of many employees experiencing impairment or illness. There is recognition in using accurate descriptions of bleeding, leaking, pain, exhaustion, and/or incontinence. Using appropriate non-homogenising language might also normalise the notion that we all have bodies that require management, create mess, and fluctuate in terms of symptoms.

References

Acker, J. (1990) 'Hierarchies, jobs, bodies: A theory of gendered organizations', *Gender and Society*, 4(2): 139–58.

Bailyn, L. (2016) *Breaking the Mold: Redesigning Work for Productive and Satisfying Lives*, New York: Cornell University Press.

Bambra, C. (2011) *Work, Worklessness, and the Political Economy of Health*, Oxford: Oxford University Press.

Bellaby, P. (1990) 'What is genuine sickness? The relation between work-discipline and the sick role in a pottery factory', *Sociology of Health & Illness*, 12(1): 47–68.

Bonaccio, S., Connelly, C.E., Gellatly, I.R., Jetha, A. and Martin Ginis, K.A. (2020) 'The participation of people with disabilities in the workplace across the employment cycle: Employer concerns and research evidence', *Journal of Business and Psychology*, 35(2): 135–58.

Bramwell, D. L., Sanders, C., Rogers, A., Coffey, M. and Makrides, L. (2016) 'A case of tightrope walking: An exploration of the role of employers and managers in supporting people with long-term conditions in the workplace', *International Journal of Workplace Health Management*, 9: 238–50.

Brown, J.S. and Rawlinson, M.E. (1977) 'Sex differences in sick role rejection and in work performance following cardiac surgery', *Journal of Health and Social Behavior*, 18(3): 276–92.

British Medical Association (2019) 'Failing a generation: Delays in waiting times from referral to diagnostic assessment for autism spectrum disorder', *BMA*, [online], Available from: https://www.bma.org.uk/media/2056/autism-briefing.pdf [Accessed 13 November 2023].

Ekerdt, D.J. (1986) 'The busy ethic: Moral continuity between work and retirement', *The Gerontologist*, 26(3): 239–44.

Charmaz, K. (2000) 'Experiencing chronic illness', in G. Albrecht, R. Fitzpatrick and S. Scrimshaw (eds), *Handbook of Social Studies in Health and Medicine*, London: Sage Publications, pp 277–92.

Endometriosis UK (2023) 'It takes an average of 7.5 years to get a diagnosis of endometriosis – it shouldn't', *Endometriosis UK*, [online], Available from: https://www.endometriosis-uk.org/it-takes-average-75-years-get-diagnosis-endometriosis-it-shouldnt [Accessed 21 November 2023].

Foster, D. (2007) 'Legal obligation or personal lottery? Employee experiences of disability and the negotiation of adjustments in the public sector workplace', *Work, Employment & Society*, 21: 67–84.

Frayne, D. (2015) *The Refusal of Work: The Theory and Practice of Resistance to Work*, London: Bloomsbury Publishing.

Gavin, N.T. (2021) 'Below the radar: A UK benefit fraud media coverage tsunami – Impact, ideology, and society', *The British Journal of Sociology*, 72(3): 707–24.

Gerhardt, U. (1979) 'The Parsonian paradigm and the identity of medical sociology', *The Sociological Review*, 27(2): 229–50.

Gignac, M.A., Bowring, J., Jetha, A., Beaton, D.E., Breslin, F.C., Franche, R.L. et al (2021) 'Disclosure, privacy and workplace accommodation of episodic disabilities: Organizational perspectives on disability communication-support processes to sustain employment', *Journal of Occupational Rehabilitation*, 31(1): 153–65.

Goffman, E. (1963) *Stigma: Notes on the Management of Spoiled Identity*, New York: Penguin.

Gould, R., Mullin, C., Parker Harris, S. and Jones, R. (2022) 'Building, sustaining and growing: Disability inclusion in business', *Equality, Diversity and Inclusion: An International Journal*, 41(3): 418–34.

Grunfeld, E.A., Drudge-Coates, L., Rixon, L., Eaton, E. and Cooper, A.F. (2013) '"The only way I know how to live is to work": A qualitative study of work following treatment for prostate cancer', *Health Psychology*, 32: 75–82.

Handler, J.F. (2003) 'Social citizenship and workfare in the US and Western Europe: From status to contract', *Journal of European Social Policy*, 13(3): 229–43.

Johnson, H.M. (1972) 'Parsons, *The System of Modern Societies*', Book review, *Social Science Quarterly*, 53(1): 176.

Karren, R. and Sherman, K. (2012) 'Layoffs and unemployment discrimination: A new stigma', *Journal of Managerial Psychology*, 27(8): 848–63.

Kassebaum, G.G. and Baumann, B.O. (1965) 'Dimensions of the sick role in chronic illness', *Journal of Health and Human Behavior*, 6: 16–27.

Kennedy, F., Haslam, C., Munir, F. and Pryce, J. (2007) 'Returning to work following cancer: A qualitative exploratory study into the experience of returning to work following cancer', *European Journal of Cancer Care*, 16(1): 17–25.

Larkin, P.M. (2011) 'Incapacity, the labour market and social security: Coercion into "positive" citizenship', *The Modern Law Review*, 74(3): 385–409.

Nettleton, S. (2006) '"I just want permission to be ill": Towards a sociology of medically unexplained symptoms', *Social Science & Medicine*, 62(5): 1167–78.

Parsons, T. (1951) 'Illness and the role of the physician: A sociological perspective', *American Journal of Orthopsychiatry*, 21(3): 452–60.

Parsons, T. (1975) 'The sick role and the role of the physician reconsidered', *The Milbank Memorial Fund Quarterly. Health and Society*, 53(3): 257–78.

Patrick, R. (2012) 'Work as the primary "duty" of the responsible citizen: A critique of this work-centric approach', *People, Place & Policy Online*, 6(1).

Pilkington, A. (2020) 'Promoting race equality and supporting ethnic diversity in the academy: The UK experience over two decades', in G. Crimmins (ed), *Strategies for Supporting Inclusion and Diversity in the Academy: Higher Education, Aspiration and Inequality*, London: Palgrave Macmillan, pp 29–48.

Radley, A. (1994) *Making Sense of Illness: The Social Psychology of Health and Disease*, London: Sage.

Reid, E. (2015) 'Embracing, passing, revealing, and the ideal worker image: How people navigate expected and experienced professional identities', *Organization Science*, 26(4): 997–1017.

Remnant, J. (2017) 'Who gets what? Negotiating work and welfare after a cancer diagnosis', Unpublished PhD thesis, Newcastle University.

Remnant, J. (2019) 'Getting what you deserve: How notions of deservingness feature in the experiences of employees with cancer', *Social Science and Medicine*, 237(September): 112447.

Remnant, J. (2021) 'Managing cancer in contemporary workforces: How employees with cancer and line managers negotiate post-diagnosis support in the workplace', *Employee Relations*, 44(1): 229–43.

Remnant, J. (2022) 'Managing cancer in contemporary workforces: How employees with cancer and line managers negotiate post-diagnosis support in the workplace', *Employee Relations: The International Journal*, 44(1): 229–43.

Remnant, J. Sang, K., Myhill, K., Calvard, T., Chowdhry, S. and Richards, J. (2022) 'Working it out: Will the improved management of leaky bodies in the workplace create a dialogue between medical sociology and disability studies?', *Sociology of Health and Illness*, 45(6): 1276–99.

Remnant, J. Sang, K., Calvard, T., Richards, J. and Babajide, O. (2024) 'Exclusionary logics: Constructing disability and disadvantaging disabled academics in the neoliberal university', *Sociology*, 58(1): 23–44.

Rozali, N., Abdullah, S., Ishak, S.I.D., Azmi, A.A. and Akhmar, N.H. (2017) 'Challenges faced by people with disability for getting jobs: Entrepreneurship solution for unemployment', *International Journal of Academic Research in Business and Social Sciences*, 7(3): 333–39.

Sainsbury, R. (2018) 'Labour market participation of persons with disabilities – how can Europe close the disability employment gap?', in G. Wansin, F. Welti and M. Schäfers (eds), *The Right to Work for Persons with Disabilities: International Perspectives*, Baden-Baden: Nomos Verlagsgesellschaft, pp 135–54.

Sang, K., Powell, A., Finkel, R. and Richards, J. (2015) '"Being an academic is not a 9–5 job": Long working hours and the "ideal worker" in UK academia', *Labour and Industry: A Journal of the Social and Economic Relations of Work*, 25(3): 235–49.

Sang, K., Calvard, T. and Remnant, J. (2021) 'Disability and academic careers: Using the social model to reveal the role of human resource management practices in creating disability', *Work, Employment and Society*, 36(4): 722–40.

Sang, K., Remnant, J., Calvard, T. and Myhill, K. (2021) 'Blood work: Managing menstruation, menopause and gynaecological health conditions in the workplace', *International Journal of Environmental Research and Public Health*, 18(4): 1951.

Shakespeare, T. (2006) 'The social model of disability', in L.J. Davis (ed), *The Disability Studies Reader* (2nd edn), London: Routledge, pp 197–204.

Tompa, E., Samosh, D. and Santuzzi, A.M. (2022) 'The benefits of inclusion: Disability and work in the 21st century', *Equality, Diversity and Inclusion: An International Journal*, 41(3): 309–17.

Tyler, I. (2020) *Stigma: The Machinery of Inequality*, London: Zed Books.

UK National Archives (n.d.) 'Disability history', *The National Archives*, [online], Available from: https://www.nationalarchives.gov.uk/help-with-your-research/research-guides/disability-history/ [Accessed 12 April 2023].

Oorschot, W.V. (2000) 'Who should get what, and why? On deservingness criteria and the conditionality of solidarity among the public', *Policy & Politics*, 28(1): 33–48.

Van Oorschot, W. and Roosma, F. (2017) 'The social legitimacy of targeted welfare and welfare deservingness', in W. van Oorschot, F. Roosma, B. Meuleman and T. Reeskens (eds), *The Social Legitimacy of Targeted Welfare: Attitudes of Welfare Deservingness*, London: Edward Elgar Publishing, pp 3–34.

Varul, M.Z. (2010) 'Talcott Parsons, the sick role and chronic illness', *Body and Society*, 16(2): 72–94.

Wells, M., Williams, B., Firnigl, D., Lang, H., Coyle, J., Kroll, T. and MacGillivray, S. (2013) 'Supporting "work-related goals" rather than "return to work" after cancer? A systematic review and meta-synthesis of 25 qualitative studies', *Psycho-oncology*, 22(6): 1208–19.

Williams, S.J. (2005) 'Parsons revisited: from the sick role to …?', *Health*, 9(2): 123–44.

10

Spoiled Identity and the Curated Self: Narrativising Stigma in Parents' Memoirs of Raising Disabled Children

Harriet Cooper

Introduction

This chapter examines the negotiation of disability-related stigma in 21st-century Anglo-American memoir culture. How, it asks, do parents deploy a life-narrative approach to negotiate a perceived spoiled identity arising out of the arrival of a disabled child in their lives? I argue that the possibilities of self-curated social media technologies and the related ecology of the memoir industry offer opportunities to narrativise parenthood differently, aimed at taking account of and resignifying a perceived loss associated with the stigma of disability. Moreover, as theorists of memoir and disability including Apgar (2023) and Couser (2004) have argued, the production of memoir allows privileged parents to recuperate the social and reputational capital whose loss is associated with the devalued personhood of the disabled child. I explore some of the challenges and opportunities afforded by memoir culture to the representation of disability-related stigma.

Parental memoirs reveal that the disabled child's arrival is experienced as requiring a 'story'; childhood disability seems to need explaining. There is, therefore, an intimate connection between stigma, temporality, and narrative. Further, a focus on the 21st-century cultural production of narrativised selves in life-writing – and on the uneven availability of the memoir industry to different actors with a 'disability story' – gives us insight into the limitations of both the memoir form and the interactionist idea of a 'spoiled identity' (Goffman, 1963) for an inclusive political economy of disability-related stigma. To develop this argument, I use Puar's (2017) concept of 'debility' as a term that reveals the dominance of a mode of thinking about disability that positions it as 'the exception'. I also draw on Berlant's (2008) discussion of the strange fate of politics in 'sentimental' literary genres, including memoir, to propose that contemporary entrepreneurial modes of cultural self-production hinder the emergence of a more transformative and macrosocial concept of stigma. The social studies of stigma must – I suggest – attend to the political economy of cultural production to progress in the 21st century.

I critique a culture that makes it necessary to recuperate an identity 'spoiled' by the arrival of disability, rather than seeking to critique individual memoirs per se, or what they articulate. My critique is not so much of memoir culture itself, but, more precisely, of a disabling neoliberal cultural conjuncture that necessitates practices of self-curation through memoir and other similar vehicles. As I will show, 21st-century parental memoir culture has the potential to reinforce a normative narrative of child development that re-entrenches both Whiteness as normativity and disability-related stigma (Piepmeier, 2012; Apgar, 2023).

I begin by reviewing key ideas from stigma studies that inform this chapter, and by setting out a working definition of stigma. From here, I briefly explore how sociology and literary studies inflect the question of what it means, ethically, to handle accounts of others' lives. The two disciplines' orientation towards representations of 'real lives' has, I suggest, been destabilised in and through the cultural turn to the self that accompanies, and is afforded by, the rise of communicative media technologies. Then, arriving at the narrative qualities of stigma that are brought into play by life-narrative, I analyse passages of text from two parental memoirs of disabled children, both written by White cis women in the 2010s (Adams, 2013; Wright, 2015). One of these women is an academic based in New York (Adams, author of *Raising Henry: A Memoir of Motherhood, Disability, and Discovery*), writing about the arrival of her second child. The other is a UK-based nurse (Wright, author of *The Skies I'm Under: The Rain and Shine of Parenting a Child with Complex Disabilities*), whose memoir recounts the birth and childhood of her first child. We see how the arrival of the disabled child acts as a prompt-to-parental-narrative, with memoir seeming to provide a space in which to negotiate interactional stigma, and to connect with an empathetic readership. I will analyse these textual phenomena in relation to the cultural turn to the self, to see what they help us understand about disability-related stigma in contemporary Anglo-American culture.

Stigma studies in sociology and the potential contribution of literary studies

This chapter takes the socio-material context of stigma as a starting point – that is, the way in which stigma experience is situated within social and economic power relations. It has been widely noted that Goffman's influential mid-20th-century interactionist account of stigma does not explore the role of power as an organising force (Scambler, 2009; Monaghan and Williams, 2013; Tyler, 2020). Link and Phelan (2001, 375) point out that 'it takes power to stigmatise', while Scambler (2009) and Tyler (2020) have both argued convincingly for an account of stigma that conceptualises it as an effect of inequitable socio-material relations.

For Tyler (2020, 99), stigma is the 'machinery' of inequality; her critique of Goffman is that 'social relations are always already structured through histories of power (and resistance)'. My own interest here is precisely in these histories of power that Tyler highlights; how do they make themselves felt when disability 'arrives' in the life of a parent of a disabled child? Starting with a materialist concept of stigma, which recognises that stigma arises within a network of unequal class and power relations, I will consider how the stigma surrounding the figure of the disabled child in our contemporary cultural conjuncture can be better understood by engaging with its temporal and narrative qualities. This stigma comes about in the context of cultural narratives about disability (Apgar, 2023). Crafting a story about a disabled child is – I argue – a way of seeking to negotiate a way through stigmatisation, for the parents of that child. It is also an activity that is expected of parents in this situation, as we shall see (Adams, 2013). Thus, this chapter conceptualises stigma as an experience of spoiled identity that is always already situated within existing histories of power, as well as within narrative relations that structure the interactional form stigma comes to take.

The narrative aspects of stigma experience have been understudied, although Williams and Annandale's (2020, 432) analysis of the 'expectation' of weight gain, and its linkage with perceived individual 'ill-discipline', opens avenues around the narration of stigmatised experience. Regarding one participant's discourse on the anticipation of weight gain, Williams and Annandale (2020, 432) argue: 'Here, predicting weight-gain is a form of confessional designed to protect self-esteem'. There is an anticipatory temporality around stigma, with prediction playing a role in impression management. Elsewhere, disability theorists Healey and Titchkosky (2022) have described their own response to their disability-related, self-perceived 'non-normative' social practices as 'self-stigmatising'. They stigmatise *themselves* and *their* modes of engaging with the world *post-hoc*, to achieve a phantom normalcy that restores a social order. Thus, we see that the work of managing stigma is temporal and narrative work.

The arguments of Healey and Titchkosky (2022) build on Goffman's notion of 'phantom acceptance' – that is, the idea that the stigmatised individual is expected to act 'so as to imply neither that [their] burden is heavy nor that bearing it has made [them] different from us' (Goffman, 1963, 147). As we see later in the chapter, this concept can be useful for analysing parents' accounts of painful interactions with other parents whose children are 'normal'. Yet, an idea of an inauthentic (or phantom) mode of relating is also what parents may ostensibly *reject* in writing their memoirs. A key feature of contemporary self-curatorial culture is the perceived 'authentic' relation that the memoirist can cultivate with an intimate public (Berlant, 2008). The memoir thus appears, invitingly, as a site in which it becomes possible to break through stigma, to make stigma 'public' and thereby to heal the 'heavy burden' that historically had to be borne by the individual. However, as we shall see, this healing work is not entirely achievable at a social-structural level via the vehicle of memoir. The entanglement of the memoir form with extractive, capitalist social relations constrains its potential to move beyond an interactionist concept of stigma and towards a socio-material approach.

We can think of contemporary parental memoir as a genre that both manifests and produces contemporary social relations (Grossberg, 2010), a perspective which is common in the field of cultural studies. I will argue, drawing on the work of Berlant (2008) and Puar (2017), that the generic conventions of life-writing move us back towards individualist conceptualisations of disability-related stigma, in which stigma is seen as something that must be grappled with and overcome. This conceptualisation leaves us with the question of who gets to be the subject of stigma, and whose life reaches a threshold of visibility that makes it a convincing subject for memoir.

Ethical prisms and layers: working with others' accounts in sociology and literary studies

As a scholar who began in literary studies and moved into medical sociology to pursue a second doctorate, I have been struck by the fields' divergent disciplinary approaches to the question of how to analyse a text. Crudely, sociology and literary studies have historically been distinguished by their texts' respective orientations towards an 'out-there' reality. Disciplinary distinctions have historically arisen that position the object of literary studies as 'fictional' material, while the domains of sociology and history have been understood to focus on 'real lives' (Williams, 1977). The field of literary studies operates, by convention, in the domain of aesthetic analysis and interpretation, while sociology is faced with the question of what might be at stake, ethically, in attending to the aesthetic or affective qualities of a text that 'belongs' to someone else – usually to someone who is not in control of the interpretive work. While literary studies have mainly been concerned with the *practice* of interpretation, sociology has been more concerned with the *ethics* of interpretation.

Within a sociological tradition that is dedicated to observing and recording an 'out-there' reality (often referred to as positivism), there can be concern about the role of the researcher's subjectivity in the interpretation of 'data'. Yet, a sociological practice that aims only at 'listening to' and 'describing' accounts from marginalised individuals limits its potential. These modes can position the research subject only as an informant and as an object of knowledge (Chandler, 2020). Such practices can be objectifying of research subjects; they reinscribe sociology as an imperialist project of knowledge accumulation, as well as reinforce 'listening' as a paternalistic practice that encodes a hierarchy between researcher and researched (Chandler, 2020). Accounts emerging from qualitative research data must – Chandler (2020, 39) argues – be 'theorised and tied to broader issues of justice, inequality and oppression'. In literary and cultural disability studies, as in other humanities disciplines producing what Wiegman (2012) refers to as 'identity knowledges', achieving social justice is often a desired end. However, scholars such as Cherniavsky (2017) have queried how far cultural critique can in fact achieve social or political change in the post-democratic era.

The rise of practices of self-curation via social media and online blogging potentially complicates the disciplinary distinctions between literary studies and sociology as they have traditionally been conceived. When are life-narratives literary texts, ripe for interpretation, and when are they 'data' which warrant particular ethical protocols in order to be studied? Published memoirs have conventionally been bracketed with literary texts and analysed by critics as such, and indeed I follow the conventions of literary studies in this chapter. Yet, ethical protocols for studying publicly available social media (such as Twitter posts) continue to be the subject of debate.

Furthermore, the willing and playful online self-commodification that we witness on social media platforms underscores the limitations of disciplinary frameworks that separate out practices for analysing 'the fictional' and 'the real'. In the contemporary conjuncture, the self is called upon as a resource from which value can be extracted, while opportunities for productive and stable paid employment become increasingly scarce (Hakim, 2019). In this climate, stigma – as a source of 'spoiled identity' – carries particular resonances and risks, since the self has become the raw material of entrepreneurial activity (Han, 2017), enabled by the affordances of social media to communicate and, in communicating, create value (Dean, 2010). Indeed, for Han (2017, 2), 'the neoliberal subject has no capacity for relationships with others that might be free of purpose'. While this may be a bleak assessment of the penetration of social relations by imperatives to self-optimise, it can move us beyond an ethical binary as we turn to analysis of the memoirs. This context problematises a mode of analysis that would simply censure parents for writing such personal narratives or that would query the intent of parents who write about their 'real' disabled children. Parents are operating within a context of scarce resources, in which the project of destigmatising disability has become, increasingly, the plight of individuals.

I write as someone who is myself drawn to life-writing and auto-ethnography as practices for exploring complex and reciprocal psychosocial relations — between the personal and the political, the individual and the collective, the psychic and the sociocultural, the experiential and the representational. In *Critical Disability Studies and the Disabled Child: Unsettling Distinctions* (Cooper, 2020), I used 'personal writing' as a method of working with and against academic writing, as a mode of unsettling an academic discourse that might otherwise proceed as if it could be 'sure of itself' and its mode of critique. In the next section, I turn to two parental memoirs to explore disability-related stigma therein. I am ambivalent about the idea that my reading of these texts should take the form of an 'exposition', as if these texts do something that I — as literary critic — would not use writing to do. Both texts articulate feelings about disability-related stigma, and about the figure of the disabled child — themes and ideas that I have written about in both academic and personal modes. I am drawn to these texts because they evoke strong feelings in me. I both identify and dis-identify with the struggles articulated by each author. As someone who identifies both with the experience of having been a disabled child, and more recently with that of being a parent, the worlds of these memoirs are ones that are close to my life and to my heart.

Life-writing as a response to spoiled identity: the case of parental memoirs of disabled children

There is another way in which the world of the parental memoir is close to mine. Apgar (2023) observes that the genre is overwhelmingly White and privileged (middle class). I share this culture, identifying as White and middle class. Apgar (2023, 63) writes that 'the "special needs" parental memoir genre is enabled by the material and discursive privileges of White settler colonialism and, in particular, a White supremacist sense of entitlement to belonging'. Indeed, Apgar (2023) suggests a link between this sense of entitlement and the narrative of 'overcoming' impairment that is so dominant in these memoirs (Clare, 2015). The genre is predicated on a notion that 'things were not supposed to be this way for the White settler' (Apgar, 2023, 62). The response to spoiled identity that we see in the memoirs is a response that happens within a wider context of privilege. I have chosen to focus here on a US-based memoir and a UK-based memoir partly because they represent two somewhat different social and cultural milieux, and, as we shall see, in some senses, the texts counterpoint each other in terms of how they represent the stigma of the disabled child's arrival. I read both texts soon after becoming a parent myself and as I began to experience the child's 'arrival' through the lens of parenthood. Previously, I had written of this arrival from my perspective as a disabled adult, reflecting on how her own arrival in the world and diagnosis with a physical impairment might have become imbued with meaning.

'How could this happen?' The disabled child's arrival as a prompt to narrate

Parental memoirs of disabled children can be read as responding to an experience of 'spoiled identity' that arises when the 'personhood' of a child is called into question via the arrival of disability. 'We live in a society that equates personhood with self-possession, autonomy and the ability to reason', writes Rachel Adams (2013, 107), the New York-based author of *Raising Henry: A Memoir of Motherhood, Disability and Discovery*. Writing from the dual perspective of being a disability studies academic and a parent of a child with Down syndrome, Adams writes with critical attention to the specificity of stigma linked with Down syndrome, including (although Adams does not use this term) the 'courtesy stigma' – the extension of the effects of stigma into the lives of those close to the stigmatised individual (Goffman, 1963) – it may entail for parents. Down syndrome stigma could be understood to intensify in relation to the routinisation of prenatal testing for the condition in certain cultural contexts, which may then promote and embed a negative cultural idea of Down syndrome as 'worthy of detection and elimination' (Thomas, 2024; see also Alderson, 2001; Kaposy, 2018). Indeed, as Thomas (2024) has noted, parents narrativising the lives of children with Down syndrome operate in a 'curious' cultural context in which the condition is simultaneously something 'to celebrate' and something 'to screen out'.

Discussing responses to her child's diagnosis with Down syndrome, Adams (2013, 107, 108) recounts that several of her middle-class friends have asked her 'how this could have happened to [her]', citing the incredulity of a 'well-known scholar of disability studies' regarding Adams' choice not to have had a prenatal test. The unspoken assumption of the friends is that Adams surely would have terminated the pregnancy had she known that her baby had Down syndrome, as if a social norm has effectively been violated by the existence of her son. Adams (2013, 108) observes: 'Babies like Henry simply aren't born to successful, overeducated parents like us. Something must have gone terribly wrong. Many people seemed to believe that knowing what that something was would help to ensure it would never happen to them.' Here, ventriloquising these conversations, Adams shows us how the existence of prenatal testing as a choice sets up and re-entrenches the stigma associated with having a baby with Down syndrome. Testing, in this context, becomes a moral responsibility; choosing not to test is allowing something to go 'terribly wrong'. Class status, education, and, above all, knowledge of a baby's 'test-status', are supposed to ward off the possibility of disability befalling a family. Adams (2013, 108) reflects on this as a form of culturally shared common sense, noting that before the arrival of her son, she too would have been 'the one doing the asking'.

It is these stigmatising interactions that, Adams suggests, set the stage for a narrative to be told. The narrator observes: 'We live in a world where a baby like Henry demands a story' (Adams, 2013, 108). Implied in this statement is the idea that disability as a devalued social identity does not – cannot – simply 'happen' to those who count themselves among the privileged middle classes. Instead, the arrival of such a child 'demands' an explanation, to forestall the destabilising entry-in of random chance. Disability is exception in this context of social privilege (Puar, 2017). As Apgar (2023, 16) notes, 'disability memoirs respond to a shared cultural understanding of disability as unexpected and in anticipation of the question, "What happened to you?"' (see also Couser, 2009, 16). What is perhaps interesting – although not surprising – here is that Adams (2013, 107) appears to be interpellated by the stigmatising question 'how could this happen?', evidenced by the very existence of *Raising Henry*. However, the account Adams gives in the memoir refuses the terms of the narrative set up by the 'how could this happen?' question and the spoiled identity it implies. *Raising Henry* offers an alternative framing of Henry's story informed by disability history and theory, which calls into question the belief that Henry's life should be seen as a tragedy or a 'failure of medical science' (Adams, 2013, 107). Yet, what Adams' statement about the *demand* for a story reveals is the potent narrative relations within which the arrival of the disabled child is already entangled.

Within Anglo-American culture, the child's body is supposed to follow a normative developmental trajectory and to 'bear the promise of happiness', to draw on the phrasing of Ahmed (2010, 45; see also Cooper, 2020; Apgar, 2023). Elsewhere, I have written that 'a test result or diagnosis of impairment disrupts th[e] narrative of promise' associated with the arrival of the child (Cooper, 2020, 96). Spoiled identity, then, is hidden within this narrative of promise: it is its flipside, and not only this, but it is what appears as available to narrate, because the promise of happiness is a 'script' (Ahmed, 2010) that commonly does not reach the threshold of warranting narrative. The 'how could this happen?' question is the unarticulated logic of a culture that has routinised the prenatal test (Thomas, 2017) and no longer must justify it as a choice. The 'healthy baby' does not demand a story.

'[L]ittle island of motherhood': writing to unravel self-stigma

The memoir *The Skies I'm Under* documents author Rachel Wright's experience of becoming a mother for the first time, and of discovering and coming to terms with the knowledge that her son has 'complex disabilities' (a term used in the book's subtitle). The book is self-published by Born at the Right Time Publishing, and Wright now runs a podcast and website under this same name, offering disability consultancy for families and healthcare professionals. Wright's memoir explores a range of both practical and emotional issues relating to the raising of her son, Sam, from the work of organising and attending appointments and engaging with therapies, to the issue of how to find networks of support and advocacy, to how to deal with the misunderstandings of well-meaning but ill-informed strangers.

In this memoir, the '[h]ow had this happened?' question is one that Wright (2015, 117) poses inwardly, as she searches to locate a moment of deficiency in herself. While Adams' memoir theorises the way in which her child's condition seems, in the eyes of the world, to 'demand a story', Wright's book is more explicitly caught up in working through her own experience of the pain of spoiled identity. This is a text that foregrounds milestones unmet and disappointments; it poignantly and movingly addresses parental grief. In a chapter on 'Birthdays', a little over half-way through the book, Wright describes spending Sam's first birthday with her sister-in-law, her niece, and her nephew; the nephew is a similar age to Wright's son. Recounting her noting of the differences between her son and nephew, Wright (2015, 117) states: 'I wept. How had this happened? How did it turn out so differently for us?' In *Raising Henry*, the 'how could this happen?' question is posited as coming from other people, whose approach is exposed by Adams as problematically naturalising the idea that a baby is not 'supposed' to have Down syndrome. As we saw, Adams explicitly refuses this paradigm of what liberal middle-class parenting 'is'. By contrast, in *The Skies I'm Under*, the narrator poses this question to *herself*. Here is an individual searching her soul. Later in the chapter, Wright (2015, 120) reflects on what she describes as a 'mistake' she had made just before her son was born, noting that in acknowledging the 'mistake' as such, she could 'let [her]self be forgiven'. This discourse of the 'mistake' made during pregnancy chimes with Landsman's (1999) interview research with mothers of disabled children, who spent time trying to locate a perceived crucial moment or activity during their pregnancies that had, in their interpretation, led to the child's impairment (see also Cooper, 2020). While both memoirs set up disability as the exception that demands a story, *The Skies I'm Under* operates more fully within a medical model of disability as personal tragedy (Oliver, 1983) – a mode of understanding that has long been contested within disability studies, but which is dominant in parental memoirs of raising disabled children (Piepmeier, 2012; Apgar, 2023).

Stigma in *The Skies I'm Under* is naturalised as an aspect of the narrator's experience with which she must grapple. The memoir describes Wright's (2015, 169) own experience of becoming the mother of a 'severely disabled' child. The use of this phrase is described by Wright in the context of a breakthrough towards self-acceptance. Wright (2015, 169) declares: 'Like an alcoholic in an AA meeting, I was able to stand up and say, "My name is

Rachel and my son is severely disabled"'. The references here to a potentially stigmatised health condition (alcoholism), the use of the formulaic speech act associated with the Alcoholics Anonymous (AA) meeting, and the being able to inhabit acceptance in the 'stand[ing] up and say[ing]' naturalise the idea that she, Wright, has a 'problem' that she must firstly accept and then overcome. The disability-related stigma that she has internalised is figured as if it were an addictive behaviour. The metaphor reminds us that practices that are perceived to be linked to self-control are often deeply stigmatised (Williams and Annandale, 2020). Not only is disability implicitly constructed as a tragedy here, but a smoothly inhabitable parental identity has been spoiled by the arrival of disability. The narrator has frequent recourse to temporal language in this section, describing being able to speak up '[a]s the fighting *slowed*, my muscles relaxed, acceptance *grew* and I *began* my rehab' (Wright, 2015, 169, my emphasis). Here, not only does the reference to 'rehab' reinforce a connection with culturally stigmatised health conditions such as alcoholism and drug use, but the italicised terms highlight the temporal aspects of the 'acceptance' process.

As a disabled person, I find it painful to engage with Wright's depiction of the experience of coming to terms with courtesy stigma in terms of addiction rehabilitation, yet I also recognise this as a culturally dominant trope. Indeed, Apgar (2023, 41, 84) highlights the commonness of the 'tragedy-to-acceptance template' in memoirs about raising disabled children, also observing that 'while parents of typical and atypical children alike may describe the experience of child-rearing as enriching, the shapes of those narratives are distinguishable by the degree to which hardship is measured and overcome'. The successful disabled person is supposed to overcome their impairment and the adversity it is presumed to create (Clare, 2015). These narratives resonate with a still-dominant medical model of disability that locates impairment in the body-mind of the individual rather than in disabling social structures.

Within this narrative of long-term struggle, *The Skies I'm Under* frequently positions the parent of the disabled child as a pioneer, isolated on a journey to navigate a 'new normal' (Wright, 2015, 53). The experience of raising a disabled child is felt to mark out Wright as different in ways that make communion with other parents difficult or impossible: '[A] different kind of solitude enwrapped us' (Wright, 2015, 55). A sense of alienation from the anticipated aspects of new parenthood is conveyed. Wright (2015, 57) describes 'avoid[ing] "normal" baby groups', even though she had previously 'loved being part of a community' and 'getting energy from banter'. The awkwardness of social relations is highlighted by Wright (2015, 57): 'Some conversations no longer flowed, but stuttered and faltered. Being around both strangers and friends became a minefield.' Implicit across these instances is a sense that stigma is shaping interactional flows. Wright

(2015, 85) is attentive to people's seeming 'need' to be optimistic about her son's condition and highlights moments when others unsuccessfully try to draw parallels with their own parenting experiences. These lead to a greater sense of isolation for Wright. The narrator describes herself as sitting 'on [her] little island of motherhood' (Wright, 2015, 87). The friends are, perhaps clumsily, engaging in practices that manifest 'phantom acceptance', whereby – as we have seen – the stigmatised individual is invited to 'act so as to imply neither that [their] burden is heavy nor that bearing it has made [them] different from us' (Goffman, 1963, 147). Yet, Wright's reassertion of her sense of isolation at these moments suggests her recognition of the hollowness of this *as-if* mode of interacting (Goffman, 1963). The memoir form becomes a vehicle for a mode of self-expression that can break free of this phantom relation; the readership is imagined and hailed as an empathetic 'intimate public' (Berlant, 2008) in whom Wright can confide pain, grief, and difficulty. Yet, as we shall see, the mode of address used in parental memoirs not only structures, but also constrains, the work of destigmatisation.

Life-writing and individualised destigmatising

As we have seen, disability 'demands' a story. Additionally – in the life-writing context – the presence of disability creates anticipation that the memoir will do destigmatising work, via a narrative of overcoming and advocacy. In this section, I develop the textual analysis of the memoirs to explore the possibilities and constraints of life-writing for destigmatising disability. Life-writing, like any other genre, can be understood as being 'coaxed' into being through specific discourses, audiences, and environments that make it possible (Poletti, 2011, 76; see also Banner, 2017). The writing of one's life-narrative does not simply 'happen' without certain ideas about the value of such writing and such self-production being in play already within a culture. Poletti (2011) highlights that a key part of this apparatus is the contemporary notion that everyone 'has a story to tell'. The notion that the arrival of the disabled child thus demands a story, as Adams suggests, takes place within a wider social context in which telling one's story publicly is not only increasingly normalised, but becomes part of a wider cultural turn to the self as a site for extraction of value under post-2008 neoliberalism (Hakim, 2019). As a parent, and especially as a parent with access to a world of writing as a mode of making cultural capital, telling one's story as a published memoir is a practice that may 'recuperate a disabled child's access to a meaningful and valued place in the social world' (Apgar, 2023, 5). It offers a route towards the revaluing of the life of the memoirist's child and a space in which stigma experience can be negotiated, and maybe even unravelled, for the memoirist.

But can the memoir form connect with wider political goals? The genre and its conventions frame parental engagement with stigma in terms of an individual narrative of overcoming (Apgar, 2023), and this limits the potential of this form to go beyond individual (or family-level) destigmatising. Many memoirs represent a *desire* for social and political change which is predicated on the awareness-raising work of the memoir. For example, the narrator of *Raising Henry* seeks to promote the rights of disabled children: 'We all love heartwarming stories of success and accomplishment. But we're far from being a society that respects the rights of people with disabilities and their families, or that readily gives them the chance to flourish' (Adams, 2013, 250). This statement connects the destigmatising narrative work of the memoir with wider political goals. Yet, we can see parental memoirs as a form of 'sentimental' writing in the sense articulated by Berlant (2008), in that they engage a particular structure of feeling about disability, calling upon the reader to admire a trajectory of overcoming, acceptance, or becoming aware. For Berlant (2008, 2), sentimental literary cultures place their confidence in *feeling*, and, in this way, they get caught up in individualised modes of being, such as 'adaptation', 'adjustment', and 'survival'. Parental memoirs that address disability-related stigma proceed by engaging this discourse of 'adjustment' and 'survival'. Life-narrative can be said to rely on a structure of feeling that evokes an ideal of compassion rather than an ideal of social justice, to use Berlant's (2008) terms.

As a narrative of what a life with disability can be, the memoir form thus re-entrenches the idea that disability is an exception (Puar, 2017), a tragedy that happens to an unlucky individual (Oliver, 1983; Piepmeier, 2012; Apgar, 2023). Even if this tragedy can be transformed through narrative into something else, and even if stigma can be negotiated and understood in this context, I suggest the life-writing form, embedded as it is in contemporary entrepreneurial social relations of self-advancement, cannot furnish a transformative reconceptualisation of stigma that makes visible the wider social context of disability-related stigma. For Puar, the terminology of 'disability' itself leads us to think at the level of the individual's story, and it is in this sense insufficient for a politics that would make the debilitations of neocolonial capitalist social relations appear. Such debilitations might include, for example, the exposure of whole populations to dangerous toxins, or to disasters made more likely by climate crisis. Puar (2017, xv) writes: '[W]hile some bodies may not be recognized as or identify as disabled, they may well be debilitated, in part by being foreclosed access to legibility and resources as disabled'. Thus, the language of 'disability', for Puar, engages us at the level of privileged bodies that are *already* retrieved for rights. In a similar vein, I argue here that while many memoirs clearly do seek to destigmatise disabled childhoods, the form of the memoir as well as the relative inaccessibility of this creative industry to those without certain social privileges make it difficult for its demands to be felt as political (Berlant, 2008).

Conclusion

In this chapter, I have argued that 21st-century self-curatorial culture offers privileged parents of disabled children opportunities to work through and resignify the stigma associated with the arrival of a child whose development is non-normative. I argued, in particular, that in parental memoirs charting the arrival of a disabled child, the disabled child's very presence is experienced as a 'demand for a story'. This form of parental spoiled identity, and its management, can thus be understood in temporal and narrative terms. Narrators find themselves invited to engage in practices of 'explaining' the presence of the disabled child, whether this be in accordance with, or against, the terms of the 'questions' they encounter. Writing itself becomes a way of narrativising stigma and spoiled parental identity, and thereby navigating it, or working to 'overcome' it (Clare, 2015; Apgar, 2023). The memoir form offers the promise of destigmatising disability and authentic connection with an empathetic readership (Berlant, 2008) via a narrative of overcoming.

I also argued that the memoir form, and the entrepreneurial social relations of the creative industry within which it is embedded, impose a constraint on the work of destigmatising that life-narrative can do. Because of the way in which parental memoirs follow a certain template, whereby disability's arrival demands a story, they also position disability as 'the exception' (Puar, 2017). The form is also governed by an ideal of compassion rather than an ideal of social justice (Berlant, 2008). The analytic of compassion-for-all might at first glance seem to be working *against* the idea of disability-as-exception, yet, in fact, these strands work together to posit a White, middle-class, privileged disabled body that more easily comes into view as the worthy object of our empathy, even as the endemic debilitation of whole populations slips away from view (Berlant, 2008; Puar, 2017). Compassion is a lens that centres the individual rather than collective. I have argued that the tendency of the life-narrative form to mobilise the reader's compassion on the one hand, and to rely on a mode of understanding disability-as-exception on the other hand, effectively maintains stigma as a concept that refers to an *individual* experience. The very 'narrative recognition' (Apgar, 2023, 15) that memoir writers can achieve for their *own* stigmatised experiences is predicated on the invisibility of debilitated others. Ironically, this re-entrenches disability-related stigma on a macrosocial level, even as any particular life-narrative may unravel some of the stigma experienced by the family or individual in question and may take up an overtly political position.

The argument I make here matters because the self-curatorial culture of our age is socially pervasive and has a powerful effect on the extent to which we find ourselves able to think stigma beyond an interactionist account. The increasingly precarious conditions under which creative and intellectual labour takes place (Hakim, 2019) are an important context for questioning whether cultural openness about disability-related stigma is the same thing as macrosocial change. Even if we now live in a culture in which stigmatising experiences can be narrativised and negotiated, a question remains about whether this culture can support a socially transformative account of stigma.

Could things be different?

- When a social phenomenon such as disability seems to 'demand a story', we can ask which other social phenomena are naturalised as *not* seeming to need a story, and how this difference reinforces stigma. If we did this, we could more easily notice when stigma is being understood as if it were a 'thing' attached to a person, rather than a social relation.
- We can think more critically about the power of memoirs, and of other media, in shaping cultural narratives about disabled children and the work of parenting them. This will help us to see how these narratives permeate health and social care settings in ways that perpetuate stereotypical ideas about what constitutes a good quality-of-life.
- Cultural and literary analysis can help us to understand how representations themselves play a role in the social reproduction of stigma and stigmatising inequalities. Better knowledge and awareness of this could improve disabled people's day-to-day social interactions, because other people will have had opportunities to reflect on the impact of the cultural sphere on how we imagine disabled people's lives.

References

Adams, R. (2013) *Raising Henry: A Memoir of Motherhood, Disability, and Discovery*, New Haven and London: Yale University Press.

Ahmed, S. (2010) *The Promise of Happiness*, Durham NC: Duke University Press.

Alderson, P. (2001) 'Down's syndrome: Cost, quality and value of life', *Social Science and Medicine*, 53(5): 627–38.

Apgar, A. (2023) *The Disabled Child: Memoirs of a Normal Future*, Ann Arbor: University of Michigan Press.

Banner, O. (2017) *Communicative Biocapitalism: The Voice of the Patient in Digital Health and the Health Humanities*, Ann Arbor: University of Michigan Press.

Berlant, L. (2008) *The Female Complaint: The Unfinished Business of Sentimentality in American Culture*, Durham, NC: Duke University Press.

Chandler, A. (2020) 'Shame as affective injustice: Qualitative sociological explorations of self-harm, suicide and economic inequalities', in M. Button and I Marsh (eds), *Suicide and Social Justice: New Perspectives on the Politics of Suicide and Suicide Prevention*, New York and London: Routledge, pp 32–49.

Cherniavsky, E. (2017) *Neocitizenship: Political Culture after Democracy*, New York: New York University Press.

Clare, E. (2015) *Exile and Pride: Disability, Queerness and Liberation*, Durham, NC: Duke University Press.

Cooper, H. (2020) *Critical Disability Studies and the Disabled Child: Unsettling Distinctions*, London: Routledge.

Couser, G.T. (2004) *Vulnerable Subjects: Ethics and Life-Writing*, Ithaca: Cornell University Press.

Couser, G.T. (2009) *Signifying Bodies: Disability in Contemporary Life-Writing*, Ann Arbor: University of Michigan Press.

Dean, J. (2010) *Blog Theory: Feedback and Capture in the Circuits of Drive*, Cambridge: Polity Press.

Goffman, E. (1963) *Stigma: Notes on the Management of Spoiled Identity*, New York: Simon and Schuster.

Grossberg, L. (2010) *Cultural Studies in the Future Tense*, Durham, NC: Duke University Press.

Hakim, J. (2019) *Work That Body: Male Bodies in Digital Culture*, London: Rowman and Littlefield.

Han, B. (2017) *Psychopolitics: Neoliberalism and New Technologies of Power*, London: Verso.

Healey, D. and Titchkosky, T. (2022) 'A primal scene: Disability in everyday life', in M.H. Jacobsen and G. Smith (eds), *The Routledge International Handbook of Goffman Studies*, London: Routledge, pp 242–52.

Kaposy, C. (2018) *Choosing Down Syndrome: Ethics and New Prenatal Testing Technologies*, Cambridge, MA: MIT Press.

Landsman, G. (1999) 'Does God give special kids to special parents? Personhood and the child with disabilities as gift and giver', in L. Layne (ed), *Transformative Motherhood: On Giving and Getting in Consumer Culture*, New York: New York University Press, pp 133–65.

Link, B. and Phelan, J. (2001) 'Conceptualizing stigma', *Annual Review of Sociology*, 27: 363–85.

Monaghan, L. and Williams, S. (2013) 'Stigma', in J. Gabe and L. Monaghan (eds), *Key Concepts in Medical Sociology* (2nd edn), London: Sage, pp 59–62.

Oliver, M. (1983) *Social Work with Disabled People*, London: Macmillan.

Piepmeier, A. (2012) 'Saints, sages and victims: Endorsement of and resistance to cultural stereotypes in memoirs by parents of children with disabilities', *Disability Studies Quarterly*, 32(1).

Poletti, A. (2011) 'Coaxing an intimate public: Life narrative in digital storytelling', *Continuum: Journal of Media and Cultural Studies*, 25(1): 73–83.

Puar, J. (2017) *The Right to Maim: Debility, Capacity, Disability*, Durham, NC: Duke University Press.

Scambler, G. (2009) 'Health-related stigma', *Sociology of Health and Illness*, 31(3): 441–55.

Thomas, G. (2017) *Down's Syndrome Screening and Reproductive Politics: Care, Choice and Disability in the Pre-Natal Clinic*, London: Routledge.

Thomas, G. (2024) '"We wouldn't change him for the world, but we'd change the world for him": parents, disability, and the cultivation of a positive imaginary', *Current Anthropology*, 65(S26): S32–S54.

Tyler, I. (2020) *Stigma: The Machinery of Inequality*, London: Bloomsbury.

Wiegman, R. (2012) *Object Lessons*, Durham, NC: Duke University Press.

Williams, O. and Annandale, E. (2020) 'Obesity, stigma and reflexive embodiment: *Feeling* the "weight" of expectation', *Health*, 24(4): 421–41.

Williams, R. (1977) *Marxism and Literature*, Oxford: Oxford University Press.

Wright, R. (2015) *The Skies I'm Under: The Rain and Shine of Parenting a Child with Complex Disabilities*, Great Britain: Born at the Right Time Publishing.

11

Studying Up: Understanding Power in Stigmatisation, Discrimination, and Health

Andy Guise, Simone Helleren, and River Újhadbor

Introduction

There is a growing consensus that we need to 'study up' on stigma and discrimination (Wacquant, 2008; Paton, 2018; Tyler and Slater, 2018). Studying up involves trying to understand how power and responsibility are exercised, with particular attention paid to 'those who shape attitudes and actually control institutional structures' (Nader, 1974, 284). That means examining how stigma is 'designed, crafted and activated' to govern (Tyler, 2020, 269). This approach is foundational to recognising what stigma is and how it impacts health. Stigma is not a fixed mark or inherent property of an individual or group. Instead, it is more accurate to say that there is a process of stigmatisation. What is stigmatised reflects ongoing social processes of some people, conditions, or places being marked out as undesirable or degraded (Goffman, 1963; McLaughlin, 2021). Such processes are defined by power and inequality (Parker and Aggleton, 2003), and we need to study up to understand how and why.

In this chapter, we aim to support others working on health and illness to study up on stigmatisation, whether they are a student, policy maker, activist, or researcher. We provide an overview of recent writing and research in this area. From here, we introduce a framework for how to think about studying up on stigmatisation, health, and illness. We describe three essential ingredients for studying up: 1) power – we need to think about what power is and how it plays out in everyday life in order to study it; 2) positionality – we need to know how researchers involved in studying up shape and limit what can be studied; and 3) practice – we need to understand the methods we can use to examine power and how to go about doing it. Finally, we look at three case studies of studying up: 1) trans medicine and 'evidence-based' care; 2) place-based stigma and urban regeneration; and 3) leprosy workers and the power of claims to stigma. These case studies illustrate what studying up on stigmatisation can bring to research into health and illness. With this framework and these case studies, we aim to provide a guide to others considering or currently studying up. However, first, we need to clarify why we need to study up.

Why study up?

There is a consensus that research on stigma and discrimination – especially as it relates to health – has not sufficiently engaged with the sociopolitical forces that drive stigma (Link and Phelan, 2001; Parker and Aggleton, 2003; Scambler, 2009; Tyler, 2020). Following Goffman's seminal text, which explores how stigma is experienced and managed in interpersonal interactions (Goffman, 1963), much research has oriented to this level (Link and Phelan, 2001; Parker and Aggleton, 2003; Tyler, 2020). This attention to the 'micro' is important because it explores experiences of stigmatisation and discrimination in detail and how they detrimentally impact health and disease, and can centre on healthcare and health policy (Stangl et al, 2019).

However, our overall picture of stigmatisation, health, and illness is uneven. The attention paid to people's experiences of stigmatisation has not been matched by a focus on the social processes and actors involved in producing stigma (Link and Phelan, 2001; Parker and Aggleton, 2003; Tuck, 2009; Tyler, 2020). For example, plenty of research recognises healthcare access challenges for people who are homeless (Reilly et al, 2022), but research rarely considers how the limited availability of adequate housing and housing support has come about *through* stigmatisation (Slater, 2018). We know about the proliferation of food banks and the shame some people feel for having to use them, but less consideration has been afforded to how austerity and this punitive regime of welfare has come about and who stands to gain from it (Garthwaite, 2016; Tyler, 2020). This is not to say that there is no evidence of studying up in ways that address the social processes and power shaping stigma and impacting people's health (Wacquant, 2008; Scambler, 2018). However, there is simply not enough (Tyler, 2020).

This uneven understanding of stigmatisation and health has consequences. One effect is limited progress on both healthcare and public health responses to stigma at structural levels (Rao et al, 2019). There is a long history of health-related efforts to address stigma through targeting individuals and their behaviour through, for example, awareness raising, literacy campaigns, training, and enabling social contact. Evidence for these interventions is mixed, with efforts often showing little or even negative effects (National

Academies of Sciences, Engineering, and Medicine, 2016). With more studying up, we can improve understandings of where and how we might intervene to make changes 'further up' where power lies, and how it may be being abused to the advantage of the few and to the detriment of the many. In this way, instead of interventions with an individualistic approach to education, we could be pushing for policy reform that targets institutions that shape public understandings and norms.

Current uneven research efforts can also make stigma worse. Health research often focuses on specific aspects of marginalised communities (for example, a lack of resources and experiences of violence) and their difficult experiences (for example, suffering and health risks). While this research is often done in the hope of learning about the 'problem' to inform health policy and improve peoples' lives, it can simultaneously reinforce or generate stigmatising labels and hierarchies (Syvertsen and Guise, 2016). It can also add to prevailing stereotypes of people as damaged, hopeless, and powerless (Scott, 1997). For example, we recognise that some of our own research on HIV prevention among people who inject drugs has done this. Asking questions of, and focusing on, the experiences of people who inject drugs generated tensions with other groups of people who used but did not inject drugs, and, in so doing, exacerbated stigma (Syvertsen and Guise, 2016).

We started this section by asking 'why study up?'. Another important question is 'why have we not been studying up more?'. While there are many possible explanations, here we focus on three main challenges: the first is the difficulty of conceptualising power and so knowing what to look for; the second is that the individuals and groups of researchers focusing on stigma, discrimination, and health have tended to hold positions and carry assumptions about the world which can limit studying up; the third involves the practical challenges of studying up, including what data to collect, where, and how, especially when those who wield power and direct stigmatisation might not want this exposed. In this chapter, we respond to each of these challenges and explore some ideas to help us think through how to best approach studying up. First, we think about power, and then use that to sketch out both the positionality of researchers and the practicalities of designing a study and collecting data.

Power

Studying up involves examining power. Power gives someone the ability or capacity to do something. Or, at least, that is a basic starting definition that opens up a bigger question of the multiple forms of power and the many ways in which it operates. There is a need for anyone studying up to carefully think about power and their assumptions about it before studying up. With that clarity, we know what to look for and can then develop a collective effort to study up and expose power. There are many concepts and theories to help think with depth and precision about what power is and how it operates – for instance, concepts of capital (Bourdieu, 1990), discourse (Foucault, 1977), and intersectionality (Crenshaw, 1991). Rather than trying to cover all possible thinking on power, we offer some foundational insights from existing approaches to studying up on stigmatisation, discrimination, and health.

Link and Phelan (2014, 24) think about how 'stigmatisers' can use stigma to keep people 'down, in or away', and relate this to experiences of mental ill-health. Here, then, some people are understood as 'up' in that they can keep other people 'down, in or away'. The vertical logic of 'up' and its opposite 'down' indicate power and control. Such ideas are intuitive and give us a basic grasp of how we could think about power; individuals and groups have different levels of power in relation to each other, and power is exercised over other people – 'up' vs 'down' – in a hierarchy. Such thinking is already common in social research on health – for example, how there can be hierarchies among different healthcare professionals, such as doctors 'over' nurses (Walby et al, 1994), and then hierarchies of healthcare professionals 'over' patients (Parsons, 1951). It is such hierarchies that enable some groups to impose particular ideas – in this case, stigmatising ideas – onto others.

Power, though, is not just a force acting from 'up' to 'down'. While hierarchies might be the main way to conceptualise power in relation to stigma, power can also be resisted and challenged by those who are stigmatised. Tyler (2020) writes about stigma struggles, defining these as community-driven mobilisation against stigma and discrimination. Chief among her examples is the 1960s civil rights movement in the US and how Black Americans took independent action against the institutionalised violence and racism they experienced. The work of HIV activists globally to counter the stigmatisation they faced and barriers to treatment is another example of this role of struggle (France, 2017). While power is concentrated and can have a clear and significant impact on stigma and health, individuals and groups can act in a whole range of ways to counter, mitigate, or quietly subvert the power and stigma they face that might impact their health.

Thinking about 'stigmatisers' and the 'stigmatised' is useful in drawing attention to where power concentrates. Some individuals and groups have considerable power to guide stigmatisation with severe consequences for people and their health. For example, the history of the HIV epidemic featured senior leaders openly stigmatising gay men to justify delayed action (France, 2017). Or, more recently, politicians across international contexts have stigmatised the receipt of welfare benefits by those experiencing ill-health (Tyler, 2020). But there is a risk of underplaying the complexity of power if we focus too much on the idea of 'stigmatisers', whether individuals or groups.

The full purpose of studying up is to recognise the social patterns and webs of power involved in stigmatisation, and how power works through institutions and across society (Scambler, 2020). Tyler (2020) uses the imagery of stigma working as the 'machinery' of inequality, and especially how it is used by government. Wacquant (2023) also explores the role of the State in understanding the power of stigmatisation as dispersed across different areas of government, and also looks at how the power that shapes stigma is contested across politics, journalism, and academia. Parker and Aggleton (2003) use Foucault's idea of knowledge systems to understand how, for example, psychiatry and biomedicine are forms of knowledge that can generate stigma.

The power over stigmatisation and health we want to study might then be most usefully understood through this sort of complexity – of being dispersed across society, of being a feature of large institutions or social forms, and many of these institutions in combination. While individuals or groups of 'stigmatisers' are powerful, we need to recognise that their power comes from being part of particular institutions or social groups. For example, the power of an individual doctor to impose stigmatising ideas is, in part, a product of their position and role in the medical profession and the history of that profession in society. Given the complexity of these systems, we can then also recognise there are many groups with different levels and forms of power across these systems, each playing some role in stigmatisation. For example, reception staff in a hospital do not have the same level of power and autonomy as doctors, but they do have considerable power to decide who is permitted access to healthcare.

The complexity of power within stigma also comes from power potentially being hidden and hard to recognise. The enactment of stigma in health and healthcare is frequently linked to overt acts of violence, the denial of care, and bullying (Stangl et al, 2019). Here, ideas of power as involving conflict and abuse are important. But power can also be subtle and less transparent. Parker and Aggleton (2003) build on Bourdieu's thinking to suggest that stigmatisation can be about the 'symbolic power' to shape culture and to influence the meanings of particular words, images, and practices (that is, various symbols). Such 'symbolic power' is manifest in how the medical profession can influence how particular identities and experiences are understood as negative and disgraceful, not just in the consultation room but far beyond it too: for example, in medicine's role in defining morally acceptable forms of sexuality (Hart and Wellings, 2002). Following this, people experiencing and enacting stigmatisation can be influenced 'without realising it', with symbolic power 'buried' in our culture and 'misrecognised' as natural or legitimate (Link and Phelan, 2014, 25). Here, stigma 'gets under the skin' and changes how people think about themselves (Tyler, 2020, 9);

whether that is the 'stigmatiser' or 'stigmatised', both can be unaware of the processes of power they are embedded in.

The ideas we have sketched out here help us to think about what power looks like and, ultimately, what we are looking for when we study up on stigmatisation. The main point here is the need to recognise the social complexity of power, and to go beyond a narrow focus on 'stigmatisers' who are 'up there'. The next step is to apply this detailed thinking about power to those who aim to study up.

What is the position of the researchers studying up?

A further aspect of power to think about is the position and influence of the researcher aiming to study up. Understanding this is crucial when thinking about what data can be collected and how it can be analysed. First, a reminder of some important history: there has been a long tendency to see health researchers and institutions as unbiased and value-free in their work (Sowemimo, 2023). Researchers in the social sciences might also, perhaps, have understood themselves as 'outsiders' due to their concern for the needs of the 'underdog' and marginalised in society (Nader, 1972). But recent decades have seen a widespread recognition of the power and position of researchers and research institutions (Fanon, 1963; Freire, 1996; hooks, 2000). Acknowledging this history brings the discussion of power to focus on the position and role of the researcher and the institutions they are in.

Anyone studying stigma and health has a 'position', whether activist, policy maker, academic, or student. That position refers to both where they 'sit' in society (in terms of the status they hold and the resources and places they can access) and the biases and assumptions they hold. Understanding this position can be helped by specific questions such as: have you been stigmatised? Have you stigmatised others? Do you benefit from the stigmatisation of others? Why are you studying up? What is your institution doing to further or challenge stigmatisation? There are no right or wrong answers to these questions. But what is necessary is for all researchers working on stigma to start with a process of reflexivity to explore their answers to them. Reflecting in this way will involve thinking about power and stigmatisation as relational and as shaped by the context and institutions in which researchers work. Asking these questions of ourselves can make the broader processes of power and stigmatisation in society visible. Furthermore, asking these questions might lead to discomfort and unease at our relative position or what we might be complicit in, and such responses and experiences are a reminder of the complexity of power that we are trying to study.

To explore this, we can think about the implications of different positions. First, let us consider a researcher with a marginalised identity, who has previously experienced and/or is currently experiencing stigmatisation.

These experiences can generate a particular insight and perspective on power when studying up – for example, a readier recognition of what power looks like and its effects, shaped by lived experiences of the negative consequences of power and a necessity to respond to it. Such knowledge can prompt particular questions and foster a particular analysis. A researcher who has not faced exclusion or stigmatisation will likely have a different position. Such experiences might not lend themselves to questions about the effects of stigmatisation, although, instead, with careful and critical reflection, would give distinct insight into the operations of power structures, from their own experience of inhabiting them. Such a position might also enable them to more easily access and blend into stigmatisers' spaces and aid some forms of data collection. Both researcher positions here are, in turn, further complicated by how their institutional setting can variously limit or enable the power of any particular researcher and how and what they study, whether in terms of the funding available (or not) or the institutional demands to do research in a particular way or to leave certain topics unexplored.

Yet, both positions will have struggles and tensions to manage. A researcher who has been marginalised might face ongoing stigmatisation while studying up and have to confront, again, problematic power structures. This is especially likely if they seek direct access to 'stigmatisers' for data collection. Conversely, a researcher who has not been marginalised might find themselves uncomfortably complicit with these same power structures through how they might be understood to align with them or, during research, not actively challenging them (Hollins and Williams, 2022). Both researchers will face struggles in managing the hierarchies of any institutions in which they are seeking to work in, and which has influence over how they do it. There is not then, of course, a 'right' identity or institutional setting for studying up. Rather, there is a need for careful reflection on what any position involves and for this to be centrally considered while designing and implementing a study.

In acknowledging this complexity of position, it is clear that studying up needs to be done from multiple positions and perspectives, potentially within one study but certainly across a collective effort to study up. While recognising this, it is also clear that some experiences and identities have been marginalised in research to date. Indeed, while being involved in any research is to some extent a mark of privilege and position of power, there is the crucial distinction of life experiences prior to this, hierarchies within academia (both within and between disciplines and institutions), and the identities and experiences that might continue to generate marginalisation and stigmatisation. So, while a diversity of views can aid studying up, we need to recognise that many institutions involved in studying up are not diverse. A consistent and coherent approach to studying up on stigmatisation and health can, therefore, also lead to research aligning with or supporting efforts to diversify and change the institutions doing research. That could take a range of forms and responds – as previously discussed – to recognising the institutional pressures any one researcher or team might face. This could mean ensuring diversity of staff within one project, or of a project team studying up aligning with other groups and their work for change (for example, equality and diversity initiatives or unions).

Reflecting on researcher positionality is essential for studying up, not only to explain a study and contextualise limitations, but also to foster responsibility and action, including as it relates to institutional change (Hollins and Williams, 2022). The next section builds on this to consider how this relates to a series of practical questions regarding research design, data collection, and study access.

Studying up in practice

There is no one research approach to studying up. This chapter, so far, has described principles and concepts that we need to think with. Moreover, any study needs to creatively use these to respond to the forms of power being studied and the position of the researchers involved. There are four considerations in the practice of studying up that we consider here: 1) who to collaborate with, and how; 2) access to certain spaces; 3) what data and methods of data collection might be needed; and 4) what ethical research looks like when studying up.

While studying up inevitably means focusing more on 'stigmatisers' and the spaces and forms of power they are embedded in, such work will benefit from being anchored in how stigma is experienced. Putting it another way, any research on stigma can benefit from working from the 'ground up' (Stuart et al, 2012). There are two main goals to this approach: to ensure sensitivity to power and its effects, and to support studying up being part of processes of change that benefit stigmatised communities (Nader, 1974; Stuart et al, 2012). Anchoring studying up in this way could take multiple forms, perhaps in combination. Extending the reflections on positionality and recognising what any neglected perspectives might be within a research team could include research approaches that centre on participation (Israel et al, 2013). We would argue that methodological approaches that involve people experiencing stigmatisation not only yield richer data, but are more likely to have a profound impact as they foster dialogue among those who hold relevant knowledge regardless of their status as researcher.

Studying up will, though, need to pay close attention to 'stigmatisers' and the contexts and institutions they inhabit, which will mean potentially trying to access or understand particular places and people. In many health-related studies, recruitment of research participants is complex. Studying those in power is further complicated by how there are often, literally, guards, security gates, and public relations experts in the way (Gusterson, 1997). People may also simply not want to be studied and to talk to researchers, reflecting efforts to conceal their power. Access to such elites and elite spaces can be helped by several strategies. As previously discussed, particular identities and experiences can smooth access. This might extend to efforts to manage identity and presentation, with styles of dress and manner of presentation that give cues of privilege potentially enabling access (Lillie and Ayling, 2021), including being associated with a prestigious institution (Aberback and Rockman, 2002). Access is especially helped by researchers holding current or previous roles and positions in the setting being studied, thereby being an 'insider' (Gusterson, 1997; Lillie and Ayling, 2021). Covert work is also possible, although ethically challenging given institutional research codes (Gusterson, 1997), and while it might manage some aspects of reluctance to be studied, it will likely not sidestep all barriers to researcher access.

Considering the logistical and ethical difficulties of accessing some people and places raises the question of precisely what data needs to be collected, and especially whether direct access to elites is needed. Gaining direct access to interview or observe elites can be valuable for understanding stigmatisation. It can shed light on certain norms or expressions of power by grounding them in the everyday meanings and contexts in which they come about. But are these forms of data essential? Data from such closed settings is likely fascinating, but insightful research can be done in other ways. Interviewing the people who are around elites and 'stigmatisers' may be much easier and also reveal less public and unrehearsed narratives. Talking with the people who work at the bars and restaurants where people with power congregate, or people who clean their houses or who service their cars, are all ways in which the meanings and motivations of the powerful might be understood (Knowles, 2022).

There are also many secondary data sources offering proxies for interview data. Newspaper interviews, social media posts, public speeches, court proceedings, tax returns, and government inquiries all provide traces of discourse. While these are 'public accounts' and so might be sanitised narratives, so too are interviews offered up directly to a researcher. Considering multiple methods, and especially strategies of institutional ethnography (Smith, 2005) which bring together different sources of data, is also valuable in exploring more hidden aspects of power and making pragmatic use of what data is available. Thinking widely on possible methods is, then, a useful response to thinking of the many ways in which different researcher positions can be accommodated as strengths in studying up.

As is clear in this chapter, there are multiple tensions in navigating power when studying up, and this extends to meeting conventional institutional research ethics codes. Conventional ethical codes for research assume participants need protecting from a powerful researcher, and primacy is given to principles of protecting and maintaining participants' wishes (Lillie and Ayling, 2021). If, however, studying up aims to expose power, and participants are very powerful, there is a different question of whether it is more ethical to *not* protect participants' wishes and whether ethical research in 'elite studies' actually requires breaking conventional research ethics principles (Lillie and Ayling, 2021). For example, we might go against participants' wishes to maintain anonymity as this might undermine the imperative to reveal power, and instead act in a broader sense of ethics in terms of the interests of equality and justice (Lillie and Ayling, 2021). Such dilemmas might present themselves in specific contexts of studying up: for example, studying prominent groups where anonymity is almost impossible. In these very specific situations, a researcher needs to carefully consider their position, and approach, and might well be ultimately limited by institutional norms. And yet, acute ethical dilemmas are likely rare when studying up on stigmatisation and health. Tensions arise over anonymity when direct access to participants is needed and so when anonymity and confidentiality might need to be assured. It might be that studying up can be done with what is already publicly available, or easily done anonymously.

By considering power, positionality, and a series of crucial practical questions, the chapter has set out a set of ideas and principles to support studying up. In the final section, we illustrate how these look in practice.

Case studies of studying up

Our focus now turns to three case studies that have studied up on stigmatisation, discrimination, and health: 1) trans medicine and 'evidence-based' care; 2) place-based stigma and urban regeneration; and 3) leprosy workers and the power of claims to stigma. We chose these case studies after looking for research projects that inspired us and helped us to think through the issues we have faced when studying up. Through a summary of each study, we draw out the specific implications for thinking about power, positionality, and the practicalities of studying up.

Trans medicine and 'evidence-based' care

stef shuster (2021) shifts sociological attention from the experiences of discrimination that trans people face in healthcare settings to the mechanisms within the medical profession that result in unfair treatment. Medical discourses can appear objective and neutral, organised into a set of diagnostic categories, neat medical decision-making guides, or official treatment pathways. In analysing how these discourses emerged, shuster highlights the numerous stigmatising assumptions embedded within them and, in so doing, reveals how these assumptions lead to discrimination in the present day.

shuster interviewed healthcare providers, conducted archival research into clinicians' correspondence with patients, and observed trans-related medical conferences across the US. Through this research, they demonstrate how social stigma around trans identities was gradually translated into supposedly evidence-based care and has been enshrined in diagnostic manuals and medical guidance since the 1960s. Rather than responding to rigorous research and analysis, evidence-based clinical pathways can, instead, be traced to the views of specific personalities and how they emerge in a contest for authority among a small group of clinicians. shuster shows how this can be evidenced through letters between physicians and particular discussions at conferences, where norms and stereotypes were gradually enshrined in treatment pathways.

These processes demonstrate how cisgenderism has shaped manuals determining treatment pathways. Cisgenderism reflects norms whereby there are only two genders or sexes that are valid and valued (man/woman and male/female). Any identities or behaviours that exist in-between, outside of, or beyond this binary are erased, diminished, and discriminated against (Riggs et al, 2019). For example, if someone was assigned male status at birth and sought gender affirming treatment from a gender clinician in the US in the 1960s, they were assumed to want to take up a stereotypical female role in society and eventually to undergo a so-called full biological transition (shuster, 2021). However, not all trans people identify with a binary gender, and not all trans people wish to take on binary gender roles (Matsuno and Budge, 2017). shuster illustrates how any deviation from the medical conceptualisation of transness, transitioning, and related treatment pathways could have resulted in patients being denied treatment altogether. To access treatment, trans patients therefore conformed to a hetero- and trans-normative narrative, inadvertently reinforcing a binary model of care. However, if trans people – in trying to ensure that they could access care – were found to be adjusting their narrative in accordance with what was expected of them to demonstrate their 'transness', they were often stereotyped as untrustworthy, tricksters, and liars.

shuster's study in the US shows how experiences of discrimination today emerge from a long-running cisnormative pathologising medical practice. The power of the medical profession to impose a cisnormative understanding of transness means that trans healthcare design, delivery, and access reinforces structural discrimination towards trans patients to this very day. Stigmatisation is, thus, entwined with the widely distributed processes and institutions of medical authority, and studying up here shows how particular groups, and medicine as a profession, had the power and authority to define, in significant ways, what transness is and how medicine should respond to it.

Place-based stigma and urban regeneration

Paton et al's (2017) study of the 2014 Commonwealth Games in Glasgow, UK, found that the regeneration and improvements to health and wellbeing for Glasgow communities that were promised by local authorities in the bid to host the games were not realised. Instead, driven by a process of stigmatisation, there was displacement and devaluation of the communities where the games took place (Paton, 2018). The context for the study was the historical poverty and stigmatisation of the East End of Glasgow. The East End of Glasgow has been long characterised by the poor health of people living there; health statistics document the 'Shettleston man', whose life expectancy is 14 years below the UK average (Paton et al, 2017). While poverty and ill-health are challenges, in the bidding and planning processes, these were documented and presented in often exaggerated and stigmatised ways to argue that the games would help the area. Official government strategies emphasised how the games could 'raise aspirations' and 'drive achievement', positioning the challenges for the East End as those of low aspirations and limited achievement. Government strategies also claimed that the public money would drive private investment that would 'trickle down' and benefit these communities.

These government strategies overlapped with stigmatising media discourses that exaggerated statistics about the number of people 'pampered' by receiving benefits (Paton, 2018). The games, while funded by public money, were then implemented through a range of policies supporting key business interests. Money for regeneration was diverted to high salaries and payouts for local leaders and politicians (Paton, 2018). Residents' homes and care services were demolished to make way for temporary facilities, with minimal compensation as a consequence of the active stigmatisation of the area reducing land values, while adjacent land owned by property developers was bought by the government agencies at much higher prices (Paton, 2018). Rather than local communities benefitting from the games, Paton et al (2017) demonstrate how they experienced displacement and further stigmatisation. The study highlights how long-running stigmatisation was then further driven, especially by government agencies, to pursue processes of urban regeneration that benefitted developers and private businesses, but not the local communities as claimed, despite the rhetoric of benefits.

Crucial to Paton's project was access to data collected by the 'Glasgow Games Monitor', a group of volunteers, including locals, activists, and academics, that collated data on the movement of money related to the games, including land sales and investments. In addition to focus groups, Paton et al (2017) worked with 22 participants from the East End who kept diaries before, during, and after the games, providing rich, personal, and context-focused data about their lives, and their lives in relation to the games. The two very different and overlapping perspectives enabled the authors to study up, but still stay grounded in the specific experiences of stigmatisation that were produced. Handing over much of the qualitative data collection to local people allowed the time for narratives to unfold from the games. The methods reveal a sensitivity to positionality and a conceptualisation of power as dispersed, entwined with discourse, and ultimately traceable by tracking the movement of financial transactions away from a place of deprivation.

Leprosy workers and the power of claims of stigma

The stigmatisation of leprosy has been long studied, and especially how patients can be stigmatised in communities more generally and by health workers specifically. Kristine Harris (2011) explored how stigma shapes the position and identities of health workers providing care for people with leprosy. The analysis aimed to go beyond the idea of stigma as something that solely affects the 'stigmatised' and, instead, recognise it as something relational with many consequences.

Harris (2011) begins by recognising how leprosy workers report being stigmatised, and as losing status, in their own organisations. Using an ethnographic approach integrating observation, interviews, and focus groups, Harris explores this declining status as resulting from the decreasing prevalence of leprosy, with the organisations these leprosy workers worked in shifting focus to address (now more prevalent) diseases including TB (tuberculosis), malaria, and HIV. Leprosy-focused health workers then began to understand themselves as old-fashioned and redundant, as new health workers were hired to address these new diseases and other areas of work. Harris reports their nostalgic narratives of the past, of dedicated service, loyalty, and sacrifice, and their contrasting of these with the new health workers who have different skills and approaches.

The leprosy workers' claims of being stigmatised are then, actually, understandable as part of a struggle for power within the organisation. The leprosy workers are using the leprosy discourse of 'stigma' to describe their own predicament and, through that, try and retain status. Harris' study, in turn, is helpful in showing how stigmatisation, and claims of it, are wrapped up in numerous health-related processes – not just experiences of illness or disease, but also health system reform and global patterns and institutional norms of financing. Furthermore, stigmatisation is not just about stigmatising particular groups, but it is also a process with other consequences, including about maintaining power and position within an organisation.

Conclusion

These three case studies offer different insights into the value of, and approaches to, studying up on stigmatisation, discrimination, and health. Each study shows different ways in which power and responsibility can be exercised or contested, and how this impacts on processes of stigmatisation and consequences for health. This could be how stigma is becoming gradually encoded in clinical guidelines, undermining social determinants of health, or a focus for negotiating position and careers within health systems. Who is 'up' also varies (for example, medical doctors, property developers, or community-level health workers). Usefully here, we can distinguish between 'elites' and those like community health workers who are 'up' relative to some groups, but perhaps 'down' compared to others. There are also varying approaches to how the research is done, whether this is looking historically and drawing on archives, embedding research within careful documentary analysis led by community activists, or interviews grounded in long-running ethnographic fieldwork.

As we wrote at the start of the chapter, efforts to study stigmatisation and discrimination are often driven – implicitly or explicitly – by an attempt to promote health and address injustice and inequities. The basis of this chapter is that such efforts should be supported by more research that gives a careful consideration of the power and responsibility which becomes exercised through stigma. This is not to claim that sociological research is the only or best route to challenge stigma. Much change on stigma has been achieved without social scientists (Corrigan, 2018). A sociology of health that studies up more on stigmatisation could, though, be a useful part of such processes of social change and, at the very least, give people a guide to the forces of power that contribute to the attitudes and institutions that shape their lives (Nader, 1974). This chapter is one resource to help achieve this goal.

Could things be different?

- Until now, a lot of analysis of stigma has focused on individual-level experiences and not allowed us to think about and challenge the social forces driving stigmatisation. Studying up helps us focus our attention on the structural forces that drive stigmatisation, and more effectively target them for change.
- There is a lot of existing research to build on that can help studying up. Studying up is not a new idea. It just needs more attention from researchers working on health and illness.
- Our framework of thinking about power, position, and practicalities of studying up can help those seeking to do this research. By using it, researchers can be guided to conceptualise power, think through positionality, and address the practicalities of study design.

References

Aberback, J.D. and Rockman, B.A. (2002) 'Conducting and coding elite interviews', *Political Science and Politics*, 35(4): 673–6.

Bourdieu, P. (1990) *The Logic of Practice*, Cambridge: Polity Press.

Corrigan, P. (2018) *The Stigma Effect: Unintended Consequences of Mental Health Campaigns*, New York: Columbia University Press.

Crenshaw, K. (1991) 'Mapping the margins: Intersectionality, identity politics, and violence against women of color', *Stanford Law Review*, 43(6): 1241–99.

Fanon, F. (1963) *The Wretched of the Earth*, New York: Grover.

Foucault, M. (1977) *Discipline and Punish*, London: Penguin Books.

France, D. (2017) *How to Survive a Plague*, London: Picador.

Freire, P. (1996) *Pedagogy of the Oppressed* (revised edn), New York: Continuum.

Garthwaite, K. (2016) 'Stigma, shame and "people like us": An ethnographic study of foodbank use in the UK', *Journal of Poverty and Social Justice*, 24(3): 277–89.

Goffman, E. (1963) *Stigma: Notes on the Management of Spoiled Identity*, Middlesex: Penguin.

Gusterson, H. (1997) 'Studying up revisited', *Political and Legal Anthropology Review*, 20(1): 114–19.

Harris, K. (2011) 'Pride and prejudice – Identity and stigma in leprosy work', *Leprosy Review*, 82(2): 135–46.

Hart, G. and Wellings, K. (2002) 'Sexual behaviour and its medicalisation: In sickness and in health', *BMJ*, 324(7342): 896–900.

Hollin, G. and Williams R. (2022) 'Complicity: Methodologies of power, politics and the ethics of knowledge production', *Sociology of Health and Illness*, 44(S1): 1–21.

hooks, b. (2000) *Feminist Theory: From Margin to Center*, London: Pluto Press.

Israel, B.A., Eng, E., Schulz, A. and Parker, E. (2013) *Methods for Community Based Participatory Research for Health*, Hoboken, NJ: Wiley and Sons.

Knowles, C. (2022) *Serious Money: Walking Plutocratic London*, London: Allen Lane.

Lillie, K and Ayling, P. (2021) 'Revisiting the un/ethical: The complex ethics of elite studies research', *Qualitative Research*, 21(6): 890–905.

Link, B. and Phelan, J. (2001) 'Conceptualising stigma', *Annual Review of Sociology*, 27: 363–85.

Link, B.G. and Phelan, J. (2014) 'Stigma power', *Social Science and Medicine*, 103: 24–32.

Matsuno, E. and Budge, S.L. (2017) 'Non-binary/genderqueer identities: A critical review of the literature', *Current Sexual Health Reports*, 9: 116–20.

McLaughlin, K. (2021) *Stigma and its Discontents*, Newcastle: Cambridge Scholars Publishing.

Nader, L. (1974) 'Up the anthropologist: Perspectives gained from studying up', in D. Hymes (ed), *Reinventing Anthropology*, New York: Vintage Books, pp 284–311.

National Academies of Sciences, Engineering, and Medicine (2016) *Ending Discrimination Against People with Mental and Substance Use Disorders: The Evidence for Stigma Change*, Washington, DC: National Academies Press.

Parker, R. and Aggleton, P. (2003) 'HIV and AIDS related stigma and discrimination: A conceptual framework and implications for action', *Social Science and Medicine*, 57: 13–24.

Parsons, T. (1951) *The Social System*, Glencoe, IL: Free Press.

Paton, K. (2018) 'Beyond legacy: Backstage stigmatisation and "trickle-up" politics of urban regeneration', *The Sociological Review*, 66(4): 919–34.

Paton, K., McCall, V. and Mooney, G. (2017) 'Place revisited: Class, stigma and urban restructuring in the case of Glasgow's Commonwealth Games', *The Sociological Review*, 65(4): 578–94.

Rao, D., Elshafei, A., Nguyen, M., Hatzenbuehler, M.L., Frey, S. and Go, V.F. (2019) 'A systematic review of multi-level stigma interventions: State of the science and future directions', *BMC Medicine*, 17: 41.

Reilly, J., Ho, I. and Williamson, A. (2022) 'A systematic review of the effect of stigma on the health of people experiencing homelessness', *Health & Social Care in the Community*, 30(6): 2128–41.

Riggs, D.W., Pearce, R., Pfeffer, C.A., Hines, S., White, F. and Ruspini, E. (2019) 'Transnormativity in the psy disciplines: Constructing pathology in the Diagnostic and Statistical Manual of Mental Disorders and standards of care', *American Psychologist*, 74(8): 912–24.

Scambler, G. (2009) 'Health-related stigma', *Sociology of Health and Illness*, 31(3): 441–55.

Scambler, G. (2018) 'Heaping blame on shame: "Weaponising stigma" for neoliberal times', *The Sociological Review*, 66(4): 766–82.

Scambler, G. (2020) *A Sociology of Shame and Blame: Insiders versus Outsiders*, London: Palgrave Macmillan.

Scott, D.M. (1997) *Contempt and Pity: Social Policy and the Image of the Damaged Black Psyche, 1880–1996*, Chapel Hill, NC: University of North Carolina Press.

shuster, s. (2021) *Trans Medicine: The Emergence and Practice of Treating Gender*, New York: New York University Press.

Slater, T. (2018) 'The invention of the "sink estate": Consequential categorisation and the UK housing crisis', *The Sociological Review*, 66(4): 877–97.

Smith, D. (2005) *Institutional Ethnography: A Sociology for People*, Oxford: Altamira Press.

Sowemimo, A. (2023) *Divided: Racism, Medicine and Why We Need to Decolonise Healthcare*, London: Profile Books Ltd.

Stangl, A.L., Earnshaw, V.A., Logie, C.H., Van Brakel, W., Simbayi, L.C., Barré, I. and Dovidio, J.F. (2019) 'The Health Stigma and Discrimination Framework: A global, crosscutting framework to inform research, intervention development, and policy on health-related stigmas', *BMC Medicine*, 17: 31.

Stuart, H, Areboledo-Flórez, J and Sartorius, N. (2012) '*Paradigms Lost: Fighting Stigma and the Lessons Learned*, Oxford: Oxford University Press.

Syvertsen, J. and Guise A. (2016) 'Navigating the symbolic violence of applied social science research with vulnerable populations', *Practical Anthropology*, 38(4): 23–6.

Tuck, E. (2009) 'Suspending damage: A letter to communities', *Harvard Educational Review*, 79(3): 409–28.

Tyler, I. (2020) *Stigma: The Machinery of Inequality*, London: Zed books.

Tyler, I. and Slater T. (2018) 'Rethinking the sociology of stigma', *The Sociological Review*, 66(4): 721–43.

Wacquant, L. (2008) *Urban Outcasts: A Comparative Sociology of Advanced Marginality*, Cambridge: Polity Press.

Wacquant, L. (2023) *Bourdieu in the City: Challenging Urban Theory*, Cambridge, UK: Polity Press.

Walby, S.T., Greenwell, J., Mackay, L. and Soothill, K. (1994) *Medicine and Nursing: Professions in a Changing Health Service*, London: Sage.

Recalibrating Stigma: Concluding Thoughts

Tanisha Spratt, Amy Chandler, Oli Williams, and Gareth M. Thomas

The contributions in this book challenge commonly held assumptions about the uses and outcomes of stigma in social scientific research on health and illness. Specifically, each of the chapters, directly or indirectly, attends to the (mis)uses of stigma by highlighting what is often overlooked and assumed when this concept is applied. Our contention has been that the concept of stigma needs recalibrating because analyses frequently fail to sufficiently acknowledge and attend to the significance of *both* macro-level (power, structural inequalities, processes of marginalisation and discrimination) and micro-level (how stigma plays out in everyday life and the experience of being stigmatised) factors. We understand and endorse the call for more attention to be directed to macro-level factors; indeed, social scientific research on the intersections of health/illness and stigma has previously been skewed towards (limited) analyses of personal experience. However, it is not an either/or scenario. It is crucial to understand how and why stigma is generated, but also what it generates and why. Moreover, it is important to acknowledge and explain the complexity, inconsistency, and diversity of stigma and how it affects different people.

In this concluding chapter, we highlight several overlapping themes across contributions to demonstrate the various ways in which stigma can be sharpened as an analytic concept in the study of health and illness. To be clear, our aim is not to provide a singular definition of stigma. The contributors in this book were not brought together because they all agree on what stigma is or have the same approach to interpreting its origins and effects. Our collective endeavour, instead, has been to address common shortcomings in stigma analyses that we outlined in the introduction to this book. Our aim is to push and support readers to trouble common assumptions about stigma in critically interpretive and reflexive ways, allowing them to recalibrate their own understanding of the stigma they witness, experience, study, and, potentially, engage in.

The brief to recalibrate stigma has led to a set of chapters with overlap in three key areas that merit further exploration. First, we discuss the need to comprehend the origins and developments of stigma by calling attention to its political economy. In doing so, we argue that attending to how stigma shifts, pivots, and mutates over time, and within and across geographical contexts, is crucial when evaluating its contemporary uses and harms. Second, we urge researchers to avoid applying the concept of stigma in universal ways. As several contributors in this book make clear, analyses that frame stigma as inherently bad and harmful, and as unanimously felt and experienced, leave little room for the agency or resistance of people who might reject this label, positively reclaim it, or remain unaffected (or even positively affected) by it. We reject the notion that stigma is universally felt by pointing to how small groups and communities can create, mitigate, and dissolve stigma, though this can be bounded by contexts of material and structural constraint. Although the pro-/anti-stigma binary offers certainty to those on either side, it can undermine our understanding of people's complex, contested, and varied experiences of stigma. Third, we acknowledge the potency of shame in discussions of stigma. In the sociology of health and illness, stigma and shame are regularly used interchangeably and without sufficient thought. The contributions in this book suggest that defining what we mean by stigma and shame, and addressing the potential interplay between them, is a worthwhile endeavour.

Doing all or any of this is not the *only* way to recalibrate stigma as a concept, though it is a useful start. We expect other researchers to have their own priorities and positions, and we appreciate that the distinctiveness of each project renders any attempt to propose a singular position redundant and destined to fail. Nonetheless, throughout this book and this conclusion, we challenge researchers working on stigma to consider not only where dominant (stigmatising) discourses come from and how they are sustained, but also how they are mobilised, challenged, and/or refused by individuals and/or groups themselves.

Understanding the origins and developments of stigma

Throughout this book, a common discussion point has been the use of stigma in campaigns intending to generate large-scale changes to population health and in political projects that prioritise nation-building. By nation-building, we refer to both the ways in which nations are constructed in accordance with ideas of national identity, and how that construction is often dependent on political strategies created to increase or decrease population numbers. The mobilisation and affective uses of stigma are understood as a way to produce 'ideal' citizens and populations that act in ways that are compliant with, and in service of, the State. That is, stigma offers a way of governing people.

This orientation presents challenges when it comes to conceptualising the individual *in relation to*, and as a *member of*, the State. Freedom of choice, individual autonomy, and the relative nature of agency are, under this framework, recognised as secondary to considerations that prioritise State interests. This, in turn, often fails to allow for individual mobilisations of stigma that benefit the self and/or constitute acts of self-preservation. Alternative recognitions of stigma as entities that can exist *in relation to* or *separate from* the State – as several chapters in this book make clear – demonstrate its fluctuating and multifaceted presence in everyday life. As an entity that is always subject to change and often dependent on the local contexts in which it emerges, stigma can be understood as a mobilising force organically derived over time and space. In other words, stigma should not be understood as a concept that materialises *only* from the 'top down'. Rather, it must be recognised as an entity that can *also* emerge organically from the 'bottom up' – that is, in ways that do not necessarily rely on top-down directives from the State or other ruling bodies (although may later be adopted and (ab)used by them).

Gillian Love (Chapter 3) emphasises these points in her chapter on abortion stigma. Love recognises, for instance, how abortion stigma often works in service of political projects that prioritise nation-building and promote subject conformity. In this way, stigma can be, and frequently is, mobilised as a productive force that achieves desired political outcomes (in this case, in relation to national concerns about reproduction). Focusing on the case of Poland following the fall of Communism as an illustrative example, Love describes how government-imposed restrictions on abortion and contraception further imposed a 'project of framing Polish women who do not have children as selfish, encouraging them to have children in the name of economic and nationalist causes'. 'Conversely', Love argues, anti-natalist States 'encourage or enforce abortion and contraception, and stigmatise "irresponsible" reproduction in order to curb what they frame as damaging 'over-population'.

By presenting abortion stigma as a fluctuating practice coinciding with the reproductive priorities of the State in question, Love argues for recognising stigma as a phenomenon constantly at risk of political recalibration. Abortion, Love suggests, is embroiled within a broader politic that attributes and withholds stigma in accordance with a person's divergence from, or conformity to, national norms and values. Here, the decision to have an abortion arguably becomes one that is always implicated in the lives of others, which, for many, validates it as a legitimate topic of local/national debate and paves the way for stigma. This legitimacy is, however, undermined by the secrecy that many who undergo abortions adopt in response to anticipated stigma. By keeping quiet, people who undergo abortions are both subject to, and exempt from, stigma that arises from public debates on abortion.

They maintain a close awareness of stigma, while ensuring their distance from it. Love's analysis suggests that a recalibration of abortion stigma can identify the power of the State to shape stigma, while also appreciating the agency of individuals to modulate and minimise the damaging effects of stigma (for example, by keeping abortions secret).

Similar to Love, Esmée Hanna, Caroline Law, and Nicky Hudson (Chapter 4) recognise how male infertility is often understood in relation to normative expectations of fatherhood, and how it shifts and mutates according to prevailing ideas of hegemonic masculinity. By reinforcing 'pro-natalist ideas about how having children, and wanting to have children, is natural and normal', dominant discourses about male fertility risk presenting the infertile male body as 'abnormal' in contexts where hegemonic masculinity is synonymous with fatherhood, virility, and nation-building. This synonymity, in turn, provides important insights into the significance of fertility and hegemonic masculinity in State projects that centre nation-building as a primary goal. Population control, and the biopolitical means through which it is often achieved, works in service of the State, not only through its aim of establishing national compliance/conformity, but also through its ability to generate productive work forces that facilitate economic growth. In this way, the political impetus behind stigma associated with abortion *and* male infertility can be understood as one that is primarily driven by financial capital and the labour that is required to achieve it.

Jennifer Remnant (Chapter 9) expands on this issue by arguing that, in neoliberal models of work that expect conformity and an unrelenting commitment to productivity from its workers, ill and/or disabled workers are stigmatised on the basis of their 'unruly bodies'. Remnant sketches out how work policies and practices in the Global North frame ill and/or disabled workers as not 'ideal' workers owing to their health conditions. This enactment, Remnant argues, results in workers choosing not to disclose health/disability information to their employers. This means they are disadvantaged in the workplace because their struggles remain unknown. In this way, the intended function of stigma is to maximise workplace productivity, but this impedes ill and/or disabled people's capacity to contribute at work because their condition (or conditions) makes it harder, if not impossible, for them to do their jobs. Additionally, they are disincentivised to disclose their condition (or conditions) and seek necessary support. In this way, stigma is associated with neoliberal political imperatives to assume personal responsibility for one's health. Behaviours and activities that are seemingly detrimental to 'good health' are routinely stigmatised when the perceived negative health effects of those behaviours manifest (as in the case of weight stigma, for example). Through self-monitoring and direct action, people in positions that allow it can avoid stigma by acting in opposition to those stigmatised behaviours, often placing themselves and their choices within a moral framework that situates them as compliant and/or 'good'. Their positionality within this framework, in turn, routinely constitutes them as 'deserving' of good health in the public eye, because they are seen to have actively 'invested' in it (Mayes, 2016). This is a process Kass Gibson (Chapter 5) described in relation to how being physically fit has come to be conflated with being morally fit.

For people who live with stigmatised chronic health conditions, maintaining – or, indeed, attaining – this position can be difficult. In their chapter on long COVID stigma, Hannah Farrimond and Mike Michael (Chapter 8) show how people living with long COVID embody the stigma associated with their condition. Long COVID stigma is both 'personal' and 'political', originating from a widespread recognition of long COVID as a contested condition that is reminiscent of a recent past that many would wish to forget. By arguing that those with long COVID embody the traumatic past, the ongoing (hidden) present, and future vulnerabilities, Farrimond and Michael argue for a recognition of how long COVID stigma fits into a broader political economy of stigma. In other words, through their recognition of long COVID as a condition that extends beyond the person experiencing it to the wider contexts in which that person lives, Farrimond and Michael contend that the stigma associated with long COVID manifests at particular moments in time because of its wider resonance with members of the public who are also vulnerable to it. In this way, recalibrating stigma could lend itself to a recognition of stigma's temporality when applied to conditions that are politically potent, and an understanding of stigma's mutability in contexts where its meaning and application are routinely in flux.

By studying how stigma is accomplished locally (that is, bottom up rather than *only* top down) and across time/in different contexts, sociologists of health and illness will cultivate a stronger and more coherent understanding of the nuanced articulations of stigma which impact people in different ways depending on their social location/s. Stigma can be and is, of course, generated and organised from the top down. Chapters in this book make clear the potential harms and implications of stigma implemented by, and in service of, the State. Andy Guise, Simone Helleren, and River Újhadbor (Chapter 11) make a strong case, and provide methodological direction, for 'studying up' in order to gain better insight into the programmes and mechanisms of stigma that are intentionally organised and funded by powerful people and institutions for this and other purposes. Even so, we urge readers not to let this important task dissuade them from considering the possibility of, and differences in, manifestations of stigma which develop and take hold at local levels and diverge from established norms and hierarchies.

The (non-)universality of stigma

Stigma experiences can (and often do) vary in accordance with a person's sociopolitical location and their (non-)acceptance of stigmas associated with their personal attributes and/or health conditions. Stigma is routinely understood through a binary framework that renders it universal to certain qualities or behaviours. Yet, it should be recognised as a phenomenon that can be interpreted in different ways by different people and groups. Moreover, its meaning for different people and groups must be understood as contested and adopted in accordance with local and temporal norms and values.

The common assumption that all forms of stigma are inherently 'bad' and universally felt – and, thus, must be eradicated – is problematised by several contributors in this book. They note the multifaceted meanings of stigma for people who conceptualise it outside of normative frameworks. For some, stigma can function as an enabling device that spurs and/or consolidates acts that are deemed pleasurable, desirable, motivating, or useful, *precisely because* they are stigmatised. In other words, the 'deviance' (Goffman, 1963) associated with the stigmatised act can be recognised as a source of pleasure which can work to sustain the stigmatised practice. For instance, Jaime García-Iglesias (Chapter 2) suggests that stigma *produces* the sexual fetishisation of risk inherent in 'bugchasing'. By orientating itself in response to HIV-stigma, bugchasing renders stigma 'productive' by highlighting its uses in instigating sexual arousal. Pleasure is sustained by an awareness of wrongdoing that, in turn, originates from the stigma that produces it. This reorientation challenges the negative assumptions about HIV-stigma and the effects it has on all people with the condition by showing how some people seek the condition *because of* its stigmatised connotations. By challenging negative assumptions about HIV-stigma and how it is believed to be felt by all who experience it, García-Iglesias critiques popular, and limited, understandings of stigma as inherently fatalistic and universal in its effects.

A similar move is indicated in our chapter (Chapter 6), which explores the complexity, inconsistency, and diversity of stigma and its effects, and how this reveals under-acknowledged tensions in notions of being pro/anti-stigma. Pro-/anti-stigma lobbies tend to oversimplify stigma and its effects. In the case of 'obesity', we argue that weight stigma is often detrimental to health which can, in turn, justify adopting an anti-stigma approach to public health messaging. However, we highlight how little attention is dedicated to acknowledging, let alone understanding, how and why the same stigma that generates harm can have a relatively benign impact on others and can lead some to engage in health-promoting behaviours. Rejecting oversimplistic binaries, like pro-/anti-stigma, makes discussions about stigma, health, and illness more accurate and nuanced. This helps us to better understand the different ways in which people experience, respond to, and reject stigma, and to recognise the impact of social drivers of suffering, illness, and stigma. Across each of the examples in Chapters 2 and 6 – HIV/bugchasing, 'obesity', anorexia, and self-harm – stigma operates in complex and contradictory ways, thereby producing effects, shaping embodied practice, and serving to both promote and threaten 'healthy bodies' and wellbeing.

Authors in this book have also demonstrated how approaches that demand disclosure to limit and/or eradicate stigma – such as urging men with mental health issues to *open up* and *talk more* – can have detrimental effects. They similarly offer a recalibration of conventional understandings of stigma by moving beyond a simple recognition of stigma as 'bad', and towards a more complex understanding of the limits that stigma places on the expressive capacities of those who are negatively impacted by it.

For instance, Love (Chapter 3) describes how anticipated stigma, informed by gender norms and expectations, acts as a barrier to abortion disclosure by discouraging people from revealing their experience. Arguing that abortion is often understood as antithetical to core feminine ideals, Love maintains that abortion stigma is directly linked to social perceptions of women as instinctively nurturing and naturally fecund. As a perceived inevitability, motherhood is conventionally positioned as a natural occurrence for women, which directly challenges a woman's decision to have an abortion. This, Love argues, can create a culture of shame which prevents women who have and/or seek abortions from disclosing their experiences. In this way, abortion stigma acts as a silencing device that generates harm by promoting internalised feelings of shame in relation to one's perceived deviation from gendered expectations.

Likewise, for Harriet Cooper (Chapter 10), the ability to disclose information about how stigma plays out in people's everyday lives via narrative storytelling is oriented from a position of (often White) privilege, where certain narratives are told by those who feel, and frequently are, well-equipped to tell them. As such, Cooper challenges the reader to question pedagogical frameworks that produce knowledge about stigma and stigmatising practices. Citing memoirs written by mothers of disabled children, Cooper further points to the role of positionality in storytelling which relates multiple lived experiences (both the parent's and the child's). In this way, Cooper's chapter provides a distinct way of recalibrating stigma by discussing it in relation to authorship and epistemic positionings that convey lived experiences through written narratives.

Dharmi Kapadia and Maria Haarmans (Chapter 1) reckon with a different set of questions that relate to this epistemic positioning. Through their discussion of how mental health stigma is understood by healthcare professionals and institutions as originating *within* ethnically minoritised communities, Kapadia and Haarmans convey the limits and harms of racialised assumptions of mental health and engagement with mental health services. These assumptions silence understandings of the role of racism in shaping healthcare avoidance and mental health stigma. Kapadia and Haarmans suggest that considerations of racism and power are routinely omitted in discussions of how healthcare services interact with ethnically minoritised patients. For the authors, stigma and racism need to be understood as intersecting systems of power that work in relation to each other to produce disabling conditions that inhibit those who experience them. In this way, studies of stigma require an intersectional approach that meaningfully considers the multiple ways in which different people experience stigma in relation to their identity markers (rather than, simply, assuming stigma for one 'attribute' – for example, mental health or racial categorisation).

Here, we have attempted to show how analyses that are entrenched in pro- or anti-stigma positions, and/or assume that stigma is universally experienced, are both oversimplistic and neglectful of the possibility for people rejecting or reclaiming stigma – or, even, being indifferent to it. A rejection of stigma can involve directly refuting negative beliefs about a person/group, body, or behaviour and, in doing so, can prevent negative appraisals from being felt in debilitating ways. Reclaiming stigma can manifest in movements and affirmations that ascribe positive meaning to the stigmatised qualities that a person or group are seen to possess. By turning stigma on its head, this reclamation of stigma provides critical alternatives to common devaluations and contradicts popular perceptions of stigma as a sign of a physical or moral defect. For Fay Dennis (Chapter 7), moving away from these assumptions allows us to reconfigure 'problems' (such as drug addiction) as 'ways of being in the world differently'. This more hopeful approach – of readdressing stigma (in Dennis' case, addiction stigma) – provides fertile ground for people to become accepted and to pursue and inhabit identities outside of encumbering categorisations such as, in this case, 'addict' or 'drug user'. This is not to deny the power and potency of stigma for some, or to dismiss the very real problems that certain behaviours (like heavy drug use) can cause. Nonetheless, it provides a vehicle for problematising presumptions of 'stigmatised identities' and, where appropriate, offers a way of relocating where 'the problem' comes from in ways that reveal alternative assessments of people's lives and more productive ways of limiting suffering.

Conceptualising stigma in relation to shame

One theme identified across contributions in this book is the notion of 'shame': not seeking mental health assistance on account of fears of shaming reactions from others (Kapadia and Haarmans, Chapter 1); the inability to reproduce as a source of shame for men and as a threat to their masculine status (Hanna, Law, and Hudson, Chapter 4); the distinction between shame and blame and Scambler's (2018) argument that they can be combined to weaponise stigma (Williams, Thomas, Spratt, and Chandler, Chapter 6); an internalised shame and blame for people with long COVID who may be seen as responsible for their own plight (Farrimond and Michael, Chapter 8).

However, García-Iglesias (Chapter 2) and Kass Gibson (Chapter 5) are the authors who most extensively consider notions of shame in this book. García-Iglesias discusses how some men balance between bugchasing being 'a source of arousal' and 'leading to concern and shame'. At times, stigma for bugchasing men is mobilised negatively as almost akin to shame: they fear a loss of work and relationships if their desires are revealed. At others, the stigma of bugchasing is a source of arousal and pleasure as opposed to shame and fear. Meanwhile, Gibson's chapter captures how shame is instrumental in the functioning of 'the moral economy of exercise' (how moral judgements are embedded in assumptions regarding physical (in)activity and health) and stigma as an embodied process. Drawing on the work of Norbert Elias, and arguing that people can feel shame when their bodies are not recognised as evidencing 'morally praiseworthy behaviours', Gibson claims that 'stigma and shame are as much a part of exercise as sweating and raised heart rates'. To fully grasp stigma and shame, Gibson argues, we should pay greater attention to how emotional responses regulate our conduct in relation to social norms and expectations.

While shame is discussed at various points in this book, it remains on the periphery of many chapters. This reflects the discipline of medical sociology more widely. Sociologists of health and illness sometimes use stigma and shame synonymously, and commonly in incomplete ways. Yet, a few others attend to them as separate entities, but ones that are intimately bound together. For example, Graham Scambler (2018) contends that 'stigma' can be regarded as an offence against norms of *shame*, whereas 'deviance' can be perceived as an offence against norms of *blame*. Stigma, Scambler contends, has been 'weaponised' in neoliberal capitalist culture, where the shame of being in poverty and/or claiming State benefits (for example) are reimagined as conditions meriting blame – that is, where individuals are marked as responsible for their troubles (due to 'poor choices' and 'laziness'). This pairing of shame with blame diverts attention away from structural inequities and, instead, individualises social problems and ignores failures of government.

Likewise, Luna Dolezal (2021, 2022) and colleagues (Lyons and Dolezal, 2017; Dolezal et al, 2021; Cooper et al, 2023) have written about the relationship between stigma and shame. According to Dolezal (2022, 855), stigma is usually 'inflicted silently and invisibly through the social norms and political machinations of a dominant social group', in ways that mark out behaviours, physical attributes, or situations as deviant and inferior. Yet, for Dolezal, while stigma is a useful concept for analysing healthcare interactions and the social impact of illness, it is a categorical term that is ubiquitous yet elusive. For Dolezal, this is because stigma is employed to describe a wide range of phenomena, such as discrimination, stereotyping, and prejudice, while people experiencing such phenomena are unlikely to use this term. To understand the stigmatising lived experiences of people and to provide a framework for healthcare professionals to confront and reduce stigma, Dolezal (2022, 855–6) argues we should 'investigate its emotional, personal and affective dimensions' – that is, shame.

Dolezal (2022) critiques the interchangeable use of stigma and shame in academic texts, as it assumes a connection between the emotion or experience of shame and the attribute or category of stigma. In response, she introduces the concept of 'shame anxiety', or the chronic anticipation of shame. This is similar to what Scambler (2004, 33) calls 'the fear of encountering enacted stigma'. Living with stigma in relation to a health condition, for Dolezal (2022), can involve experiencing *actual* and *anticipated* shame in ways that shape encounters with healthcare professionals or result in people avoiding such interactions altogether. Recognising shame anxiety provides a way for healthcare professionals to be sensitive to stigma and its impact in clinical settings. However, an appreciation of shame also extends beyond the clinic's walls. Writing about the COVID-19 pandemic, Dolezal et al (2021) and Cooper et al (2023) assert that shame and stigma were a key component of the pandemic, from anti-Asian racism to online shaming of healthcare workers and 'Covidiots' (we can also note the public shaming of those who did not wear face coverings, see Thomas and White, 2023). Equally, shame is not only experienced by more vulnerable populations; it can catch typically powerful actors in its net.

Based on the contributions in this collection, and the scholarship of Dolezal and Scambler, we argue that a consideration of shame must inform future work on stigma. Engaging with shame as an embodied emotion (Chandler 2019), and situating it in broader social and cultural contexts, can reveal how structural conditions of oppression, marginalisation, and inequality can shape individual actions. Similarly, Dolezal (2022, 859) argues that shame is not simply a 'private emotional event', but part of a 'nexus' prompting felt stigma as well as 'shared socio-political norms, along with broader power dynamics'. Recognising this arguably addresses Scambler's (2004) charge that early formulations and analyses of stigma and shame in the sociology of health and illness, including his own, failed to trace power and the political edges of stigma. Power is, in turn, central to shame and stigma. By recalibrating our understanding of these dynamics, we can better understand and address the interplay between power, shame, stigma, and social norms. This, in turn, can broaden our understanding of the analytic potential of stigma by revealing its multifaceted impacts on health, healing, and empowerment among people and groups tasked with circumventing stigma's everyday effects.

Conclusion

This book has made the case for, and demonstrated the value of, recalibrating stigma as an analytical concept for studying health, illness, medicine, and public health. Bringing together contributions focusing on mental health, racism, sex, HIV, fertility, abortion, 'obesity', anorexia, self-harm, exercise, drug use, COVID-19, employment, disability, and research methods, we hope to stimulate and facilitate conversations around stigma, particularly within the social study of health and illness. The chapters each offer grist for the mill in this regard, mostly theoretically and empirically, but also – in the chapter by Guise, Helleren, and Újhadbor (Chapter 11) – in methodological and practical terms. We hope that this book is read as a provocative and instructive resource, one which offers a diverse collection of analyses that ignite new and thoughtful insight into the social study of stigma as it relates to health and illness.

References

Chandler, A. (2019) 'Shame as affective injustice: Qualitative, sociological explorations of self-harm, suicide and socioeconomic inequalities', in M.E. Button and I. Marsh (eds), *Suicide and Social Justice: New Perspectives on the Politics of Suicide and Suicide Prevention*, London: Routledge, pp 32–49.

Cooper, F. Dolezal, L. and Rose, A. (2023) *COVID-19 and Shame: Political Emotions and Public Health in the UK*, London: Bloomsbury.

Dolezal, L. (2021) 'Shame, stigma and HIV: Considering affective climates and the phenomenology of shame anxiety', *lambda nordica*, 26(2–3): 47–75.

Dolezal, L. (2022) 'Shame anxiety, stigma and clinical encounters', *Journal of Evaluation in Clinical Practice*, 28(5): 854–60.

Dolezal, L., Rose, A. and Cooper, F. (2021) 'COVID-19, online shaming, and health-care professionals', *The Lancet*, 398(10299): 482–3.

Goffman, E. (1963) *Stigma: Notes on the Management of Spoiled Identity*, New York: Penguin.

Lyons, B. and Dolezal, L. (2017) 'Shame, stigma and medicine', *Medical Humanities*, 43(4): 208–10.

Mayes, C. (2016) *The Biopolitics of Lifestyle: Foucault, Ethics, and Healthy Choices*, London: Routledge.

Scambler, G. (2004) 'Re-framing stigma: Felt and enacted stigma and challenges to the sociology of chronic and disabling conditions', *Social Theory and Health*, 2(1): 29–46.

Scambler, G. (2018) 'Heaping blame on shame: "Weaponising stigma" for neoliberal times', *The Sociological Review,* 66(4): 766–82.

Thomas, G.M. and White, L. (2023) 'Unmasked: COVID-19, face coverings, and navigating dis/abling spaces and cultures', *Space and Culture*, 26(3): 296–308.

Index

References to tables appear in **bold** type.

A

ableism 157, 158, 166
abortion
  author's overview of 11–12, 52–3,
    208–9, 212
  biopolitics 11–12, 59–60, 62
  definitions of 52–3, 57
  discursive approaches to 55–6, 60–1, 62
  embodiment 60–2
  as internalised 54
  intersectionality and 57–8, 59, 62
  narratives of abortion 56, 63
  regulatory function of 57–8
activity *see* exercise; physical activity; sport
addiction
  addict identity 129–33
  author's overview of 13, 126
  blocked becoming 124, 125–6, 129–33,
    134, 135–6
  disease model of addiction 126–7
addicts *see* people who use drugs
anorexia 113–16
anticipated stigma 54, 144, 208, 212
anti-stigma
  destigmatisation drift 12, 105, 110–11,
    116, 118
  impacts of 27, 118
  mental health campaigns 109–11, 118
  obesity 112–13
  person-first language 112–13
  pro-ana community 114–16
  self-harm 116–18
  weight-loss 108
  see also pro-/anti-stigma binaries
arousal, stigma as 44–5, 47, 48, 211
assemblages/assemblage framework 139,
  142–3, 146, 149–50, 151–2
attributes
  discreditable attributes 4, 107
  discredited attributes 4, 54, 166
  stigma and 5–6

B

biopolitics 11–12, 59–60, 62, 76, 91,
  135, 209
Black people
  on discrimination experiences 28–31
  on drug use 133–4
  on mental healthcare institutions 27–8
  mental illness stigma 19, 20, 23
  on mental illness stigma 25–6
  reproductive barriers for 57, 58
  stigma struggles of 192
blame
  deviance and 106
  disease model of addiction and 126
  shame and 96, 140–1, 144, 145, 147,
    213, 214
blocked becoming 124, 125–6, 129–33,
  134, 135–6
body fascism
  author's overview of 12, 89, 97
  tracking technologies 99–100
body positivity 112
bugchasers/bugchasing
  author's overview of 11, 37, 40
  bugchasers, comments from 37, 38, 42–3,
    44–5, 46–7
  internet and 45–7
  reasons/motivations for 40–1
  stigma and 41, 42–5, 47, 211, 214

C

chronic illnesses 141–2
cisgenderism 199
courtesy stigma 4, 21, 179, 182
COVID-19 stigma 140–1, 143, 144, 145,
  148, 215 *see also* long COVID stigma

D

dementia 123, 133, 135
deservingness 94, 159–60

217

destigmatisation drift 12, 105, 110–11, 116, 118
deviance 106, 131, 211, 214
disability employment gap 160, 161, 168
disability studies 4–5, 160, 177–8, 179, 181–2
disabled and ill workers
 absence/sick leave 162–3
 disclosure 161, 163, 164–7, 209
 HRM policies 156–7
 leaky bodies 157, **158**, 169
 passing 165, 166, 167
 see also workplace stigmatisation
disclosure 132–3, 161, 163, 164–7, 209, 212
Down syndrome 179
drug use *see* addiction stigma; people who use drugs

E

eating disorders 113–14
embarrassment 88, 94, 95–6
embodiment 60–2, 94, 96–7
enacted stigma 92, 215
epidemics 36, 148, 150, 192 *see also* HIV-stigma; long COVID stigma
Equality Act 162–3, 166
equity, diversity, and inclusion (EDI) policies 156, 161, 163
erectile dysfunction 76, 78
ethnic minority people
 author's overview of 20
 on discrimination experiences 28–31
 on mental healthcare institutions 26–8
 mental illness stigma 19, 20–2, 111
 on mental illness stigma 24–6
 reproduction stigma 82
 stereotypes of 30–1
eugenics 59
exercise
 debates around 100
 invention of 89–91, 98
 sport as 98, 99
 stigma 12, 87–9, 214
 weight stigma and 94
 see also moral economy (of exercise)

F

fascism 97–8 *see also* body fascism
fat acceptance/activism 10, 112, 113
felt stigma 54, 61, 91–2, 215
femininity 58, 74
fertility
 of men 71–2, 75–7
 transgender people 57
figurations/figurational sociology 87–8, 92, 93–4, 96, 97, 100

G

Goffman, Erving
 critiques of 4–5, 175

dramaturgical self 96
 on power 6
 on shame 92
 on social relations 124, 129, 190
 on stigma 2–3, 4, 53, 71, 106, 136
 on the stigmatised 3–4, 77, 78, 165

H

harm reduction 123–4, 124–5, 135, 136
health
 biopolitics 91
 moral discourse of 90–1
 see also exercise; mental healthcare; public health, stigma in
hegemonic masculinity *see* masculinity
HIV-stigma
 as arousal 44–5, 47, 48, 211
 author's overview of 11, 36, 39
 definitions of 36
 impacts of 36–7, 38, 43
 narratives of HIV/AIDS 38–9
 see also bugchasers/bugchasing
HRM *see* human resource management (HRM) policies

I

identities 5–6, 129–33 *see also* spoiled identity
illnesses *see* chronic illnesses; disabled and ill workers; liminal illnesses; mental illness stigma; psychiatrisation of illnesses; workplace stigmatisation
infertility *see* male infertility
institutional racism 11, 19–20, 22, 26–8, 29–30
interactionism *see* micro (interactionist) levels of society
interactions, stigma and 4, 6, 7, 8–9
internalised stigma 42, 54, 144, 182, 212, 213
intersectionality
 abortion and 57–8, 59, 62
 biopolitics 59–60
 HIV-related stigma and 36, 39
 mental illness and 22, 28–31, 110
 pro-ana community 114
 of women 56–8, 212
in vitro fertilisation (IVF) 77, 78
Ireland 56, 59–60
IVF 77, 78

L

Lancet Commission on Ending Stigma and Discrimination in Mental Health 20
leaky bodies 157, 158, 169
leprosy 145, 201
lifestyle drift 110, 111
life-writing *see* memoirs
Link, B.G. 7, 62, 71, 175, 192
literary studies 174, 176, 177

INDEX

long COVID stigma
  about long COVID 141–2, 148
  author's overview of 210, 213
  gender and 149
  lineage, stigma 145–7
  narratives of long COVID 143–4
  stigma mutation theory and 139–40
  strength, stigma 149–51
  variation, stigma 147–9

M

machinery of stigma *see* stigma machines
macro approaches to stigma 3, 8, 9–10, 106, 107
  scholarship on 6–7
  see also power
male infertility
  author's overview of 12, 70, 209
  biopolitics 76, 209
  fertility/virility 75–7
  masculinities theories 79–81
  narratives of masculinity 71–2, 73–5
  silence 73
masculinity 40, 70, 73–5, 75–8, 79–82, 209
medical sociology 3, 5, 148, 159–60, 176–7, 214
memoirs
  author's overview of 13–14, 173–4
  disabled children, stigma of 175, 179–80
  privilege and 178, 180, 184–5, 212
  Raising Henry (Adams) 174, 179, 180, 181, 184
  role of 175–6, 183–4, 185–6
  self-curatorial culture 174, 176, 178, 184, 185, 186
  The Skies I'm Under (Wright) 174, 180–3
  see also narratives
menstruation 165, 168
mental healthcare
  discrimination in 28–31
  racism and 19
  research on ethnic inequalities in 23–4, 24–31
  stigmatisation experiences in 26–8
mental illness stigma
  anti-stigma campaigns 109–11, 118
  author's overview of 11, 20, 212–13
  ethnic minority people and 19, 20–2
  interviewees on 24–6
  self-harm 116–18
moral economy (of exercise)
  author's overview of 88–9, 91
  body fascism 12, 89, 97–100
  embodiment 94, 100
  movement intellectuals 99
  shame and 12, 88, 89, 91–2, 94–7, 101, 214
  stigma as a process 87–8, 89, 93

N

narratives
  abortion narratives 56, 63
  drug use narratives 134
  fertility/masculinity narratives 71–2
  HIV/AIDS narratives 38–9
  long COVID narratives 143–4
  mental illness narratives 20, 22, 24–6
  weight gain narratives 175
  see also memoirs
nation-building 11–12, 62, 207–8, 209
neoliberalism 58, 140–1, 159, 165, 167–8, 174, 177, 209, 214

O

obesity 112–13 *see also* weight stigma
othering
  contagious diseases and 145
  of HIV-positive people 38
  of men with fertility issues 72
  of people of who use drugs 125, 127–8, 131, 133
  power, by those in 140–1
  stigma and 10

P

pandemic *see* long COVID stigma
passing 10, 157, 165, 166, 167
patriarchy 74, 75
people who use drugs
  on addict identity 129–31, 132
  blocked becoming 124, 129–33, 134, 135–6
  on diamorphine (prescription drug) 134–5
  on drug use 123, 124–6, 133–4
  harm reduction movement 123–4, 124–5, 135, 136
  narratives of drug use 134
  othering of 125, 127–8, 131, 133
  stigma caused by research 191
person-first language 112–13, 157, 158
Pescosolido, B.A. 9, 109–10, 111
phantom acceptance 175–6, 183
pharmaceutical companies 112, 113, 127
Phelan, J.C. 7, 62, 71, 175, 192
physical activity 88, 89–90, 94, 98, 100, 101
policy
  equity, diversity, and inclusion (EDI) 156, 161, 163
  human resource management (HRM) 156, 157, 161, 162, 164, 167
positionality 14, 189, 194–6, 200–1, 209–10, 212
power
  definitions of 191
  hierarchies of 192
  and machinery of stigma 7–8, 9, 58, 63, 127
  of mental health institutions 26–8

219

mental illness stigma and 21, 111, 212–13
  othering by those in 140–1
  patriarchal societies, in 74, 75
  of shame 94
  stigma and 5, 6, 22, 56, 57, 106, 175
  studying up 189, 191–4, 194–5, 196–8, 199, 201
  symbolic power 193–4
  see also racism
pre-exposure prophylaxis (PrEP) 38, 41, 45, 46–7
pregnancy *see* reproduction
PrEP *see* pre-exposure prophylaxis (PrEP)
privilege/privileging 81, 113, 178, 180, 184–5, 212
pro-ana 114–16
pro-/anti-stigma binaries
  author's overview of 106–7, 211–12
  critiques of 109–11, 207
  person-first language 112–13
  weight-loss 108
public health, stigma in 105, 106–7

R

racial stereotyping 30
racism
  COVID-19 and 140, 145
  institutional racism 11, 19–20, 22, 26–8, 29–30
  interpersonal racism 22, 29, 30
  mental illness stigma and 11, 19–20, 111, 212–13
  and stigma 22, 31
  types of 22
re-integrative shaming 108
reproduction
  barriers to 57–8
  biopolitics of 59–60
  infertility stigma for women 78–9
  narratives of 58, 71–2, 75–6
  pregnancy 61
  shifts in attitude towards 80–1
  see also male infertility
reproductive stigma 57–8
resistance to stigma 10, 58, 62, 114 *see also* anti-stigma; studying up; *specific types of resistance (e.g., fat activism)*

S

Scambler, G.
  stigma, concepts of 5, 91–4, 175
  weaponisation of stigma 93, 106, 128, 140–1, 147, 213, 214, 215
self-curatorial culture 174, 176, 178, 184, 185, 186
self-harm 116–18
self-stigma 21, 41, 175
sexual stigma 39

shame
  anticipated shame 215
  blame and 96, 140–1, 144, 145, 147, 213, 214
  definitions of 88, 94
  infertility and 12, 72–3, 80
  mental health and 25
  moral economy of exercise and 12, 88, 89, 94–7, 101
  power of 94
  re-integrative shaming 108
  stigma and 2, 42–4, 91–2, 106, 207, 212, 213–15
  thresholds of 95
sick role 156–7, 159–61, 167–8
silence 73
smoking 107, 146, 148
social structures 3, 5, 6, 7, 21
sociology
  accounts of others 174, 176–8
  figurational sociology 87–8, 92, 93–4, 96, 97, 100
  see also medical sociology
Spanish Flu 150
spoiled identity 78, 173–4, 175, 177, 178, 179, 180, 185
sport 97–8, 99 *see also* exercise
stereotypes
  eating disorders 113–14
  of ethnic minority people 30–1
  pathologisation and 112
  stigma and 7, 21, 53
  of stigmatised people 5
  studying up to challenge 190–1
  of trans people 198–9
  of worklessness 162
stigma by association *see* courtesy stigma
'Stigma Kills' campaign 126–7
stigma machines 7–8, 9, 58, 63, 127, 175, 193
stigma mutation theory
  amplification/strength of stigma 149–51
  assemblages/assemblage framework 139, 142–3, 146, 149–50, 151–2
  author's overview of 13, 139
  evolution and 142–3
  lineage of stigma 145–7
  power, role of in 140–1
  variation of stigma 147–9
stigma transference 54
stratifying identities 129–33
structural racism 22
studying up
  author's overview of 14, 189, 190–1, 201–2
  challenges to 191
  ethical research 197–8
  examples of 198–201
  positionality 14, 189, 194–6, 200–1, 209–10

INDEX

power 189, 191–4, 194–5, 196–8, 199, 201
practice of 189–90, 196–8
suggestions for 202
symbolic power 193–4

T

transgender people
  reproductive barriers 57
  stereotypes of 198–9
  stigmatisation of 198–9
Tyler, I.
  on anti-stigma campaigns 109
  on Goffman's concept of stigma 6
  on power in stigma 22, 56, 57, 156
  stigma machines 7–8, 9, 127, 175, 193
  on the term *stigma* 131–2, 150

W

weaponisation of stigma 93, 106, 128, 140–1, 147, 213, 214, 215
weight stigma
  anorexia 113–16
  embodiment and 60–1, 94
  narratives of weight gain 175
  obesity 112–13
  pro-/anti-stigma binary 108
  shame and 94
White privilege *see* privilege/privileging
womanhood 52, 56, 57
women
  abortion experiences of 61–2
  infertility stigma 78–9
  intersectional stigma of 56–8, 212
  long COVID 149
workplace stigmatisation
  ableism 157, 158, 166
  author's overview of 13, 209–10
  disclosure of disability/illness 161, 163, 164–7, 209
  equity, diversity, and inclusion (EDI) 156, 161, 163
  human resource management (HRM) policies 156, 157, 161, 162, 164, 167
  ideal worker concept 156, 158–9, 165, 167, 209
  research on 157, 158, **158**
  sick role 156–7, 159–61, 167–8
  see also disabled and ill workers

www.ingramcontent.com/pod-product-compliance
Lightning Source LLC
Chambersburg PA
CBHW051539020426
42333CB00016B/2008